DISCLAIMER: LOVE'S MIRAGE This is a work of fiction, and this statement is included to inform the reader that any celebrity name(s), business name(s), location(s), product(s), and organizations that are stated in the content of this book are real. However, they are used in a purely fictional way.

LOVE'S MIRAGE

By: MoniB

Love's Mirage

By MoniB

Cover Illustrated by Isaac Brown

Cover Created by Jazzy Kitty Publications

Logo Designs by Andre M. Saunders/Jess Zimmerman

Editor: Anelda L. Attaway

© 2020 MoniB "Monica Betts"

ISBN 978-1-7357874-3-5

Library of Congress Control Number: 2020921259

All rights reserved. This book is protected by the copyright laws of the United States of America. This book may not be copied or reprinted for commercial gain or profit. The use of short quotations or occasional page copying for personal or group study is permitted and encouraged. Permission will be granted upon request. This book is for Worldwide Distribution and printed in the United States of America, published by Jazzy Kitty Publications utilizing Microsoft Publishing Software. Please be advised this book has strong language and content. Parental Advisory is suggested due to mature content. Disclaimer: This is a work of fiction, and that any celebrity name(s), business name(s), location(s), product(s), and organizations, while real, is used in a purely fictional way.

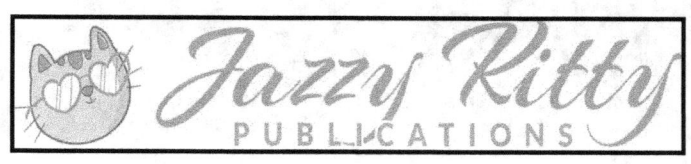

DEDICATIONS

I want to dedicate this book to my sister, Rochelle Creone. You were there doing your thing, and I took a moment just to watch. Now I see dreams can be done! Thank you so much for just doing you! You continue to inspire me.

ACKNOWLEDGMENTS

First and foremost, I acknowledge God for my writing gift and for making this happen; I truly love You!

I want to thank my mother, Mary, for encouraging me.

Thank you to all my brothers and sisters, family, and friends.

Thank you, Jazzy Kitty Publications, Mrs. Anelda Attaway, you're amazing.

If I forgot to mention anyone, please know it wasn't intentional. Thank you to all my readers in advance who will read my book; I love you all.

Thank you!

TABLE OF CONTENTS

INTRODUCTION	i
CHAPTER ONE	01
CHAPTER TWO	27
CHAPTER THREE	56
CHAPTER FOUR	82
CHAPTER FIVE	113
CHAPTER SIX	139
CHAPTER SEVEN	167
ABOUT THE AUTHOR	202

INTRODUCTION

Join me in reading what happens to Samone Grey in this epic love series. Samone Grey has a mental condition that goes untreated while amid a love triangle that goes wrong. Stuck between two men, Samone makes a choice to stick with Charles, the love of her life.

Charles is a great man, so Samone thought. She soon realizes the changes and motives that Charles has for them. Charles is the man of Samone's dreams, but she is in the middle of a nightmare.

Did she make a good choice to stay with Charles?

CHAPTER ONE

It has been five whole days since I have been able to walk outside in God's womb. I took a deep breath, and the air was so crisp and brisk that it startled me when I inhaled its scent. The aroma came with lilies, roses, peaches galore, but only in Texas could you smell this brilliance with ease.

For heaven's sake, I wish people would stop writing lies and tell the truth. Texas is a great state, but come on now, this book, well, let's just say the writer has a vivid imagination.

I threw the book back on the bookshelf and sat down. It's been 30 minutes since I've been waiting to see this doctor and to tell you the truth, I'm no good at waiting. This office should have at least two psychiatrists seeing people simultaneously; it would make it easier for themselves and leave the patients accountable for very little waiting. I'm getting anxious because now I'm thinking of leaving before I've been seen, which brings me to the reason why I'm here. I haven't been able to sleep lately, and my thoughts are like racing horses at times, so I really do need to talk to this doctor. My family probably would advise me to seek help from a psychiatrist, better known as a "shrink." My mother would definitely tell me to take it to the Lord, but little does she know my racing thoughts are sometimes about the Lord. So, I'm wondering who can help me. Hopefully, this shrink can. I need to talk to someone about these thoughts, but I fear the notion of being known as crazy or going to the nuthouse.

I waited impatiently while looking around the room. A blue-eyed woman was looking at me strangely, we made eye contact, and she looked away. She was the same woman who looked at me when I returned to my seat from throwing that book back on the shelf. Looking away, I found a brunet woman dressed in paternity clothing due to her large round stomach. She didn't notice me staring at her stomach with a smile, but I could tell she wasn't happy by her facial expression.

I thought to myself, *"why is she so sad? Creating life is beautiful; I mean, I'm actually fascinated by it. The breath of life, that is, I don't want to be suspected as being naughty, even though the physical part of creating life is equal to that of the actual act of love."* There were a couple of others waiting, but those two women I mentioned stood out to me.

I must say this doctor must be the real deal for the furnishings and decorations were quite impressive. The center table received the most attention from everyone because of its in-home peaceful and glamorous look, which triggered the couches and chairs' colors. Its bronze colored mirror reflected every inspector's eyes to see its unique style. The three-piece set of couches was covered with a silky brown covering blending so well with the tables. This waiting room looked like a set off the movies; every flower arrangement and décor was perfect. The interior designer gets an 'A' for applaud and satisfaction. While I was looking around, the blue-eyed woman walked up to me.

"Excuse me, Ms.; I was wondering why you threw that book down?"

I looked the woman in her eyes and replied, "Why do you care?"

"Oh, I didn't mean any harm; I just, well, my cousin wrote that book."

"Oh, really? That's good, but I think she exaggerated in the third paragraph regarding Texas. Do you ask everyone questions that you see with her book?"

I guess the woman could feel the steam seeping out of my comfort zone, so she took a seat across from me and gave me her dirty looks. I could have made a statement to her about her facial remarks, but I decided not to. The doctor came out and called my name.

"Samone Grey, please follow me."

I stood up and walked calmly to her office door. She stood there, waiting for me to pass her. I extended my arm to give her a handshake; she shook it and told me what she would like to be called, Dr. Givins. Entering her office, I was ready to inspect the four-star psychiatrists' classy domain in Texas. It was more than I expected. The walls were the color of sky-blue and covered with pictures of people she must have helped on a severe level. The reason I suspected that is because there was only a hand full of people on the walls, and her name speaks for many. Sitting behind her crystal top desk, Dr. Givins looked to be 35 years of age. Her hazel eyes peered at me out of those black/silver lenses that match perfectly with her oval face.

"Ms. Grey, you can take a seat right there."

I sat down in the opposite direction of her and felt the black leather seat melt with my bottom in it. Now that we were both facing each other, I realized that she was looking me over just as I was her. Her hair was curled with long layers, and the color was reddish-brown (auburn) with highlights of cinnamon bronze. I knew the colors by heart because I have the same colors in mine. I was about to ask her where she got her hair done, but I decided not to. Dr. Givins must work out because her slender size fits perfectly in her leather chair.

"I must say, Dr. Givins, you have a nice working environment."

"Thanks, Samone, but may I ask you why you are here today? I looked at my chart sheet and noticed your age." She peered at me over lenses as she gave me a concerned look.

"Believe me, Dr. Givins, age doesn't mean anything," I paused and waited for a response, but there wasn't any, "the reason I'm here is because I have racing thoughts, and I want to know how to stop them without medication."

"Oh, I see. What did your last doctor tell you?"

"I didn't ask, and he has moved to another state. His old office secretary recommended you."

"Well, how long have you been taking medication? Also, what did he prescribe you?"

"I've been taking Geodon and Benztropine for two straight months now, and he told me I could get off them in six months."

"Well, Samone, you still have four more months; what seems to be the problem?" She leaned back in her chair, crossed her legs, and glared at me. I almost felt 11 again. I sat up and began my case.

"Well, it's like this, Doc."

"Dr. Givins," she interrupted.

"Excuse me, Dr. Givins; all my life, I have been able to handle life as it has come to me, and I feel at a loss as to how to handle the medication prescribe for me. I'm not used to depending on anything or anyone, and I just want to be me without the medication."

"Obviously, you must need them. I must ask you one more question before I go on. Did he diagnose you as being bipolar?" I hated to admit it, but she was right. Dr. Lim did diagnose me as bipolar.

"Yes."

"Well, then that's just it. You need that medication to help calm or correct what was harmed in your mind." I was dismayed and vexed at what she was telling me. I heard it all before, and I knew she wasn't going to help me.

"Dr. Givins, please understand that I'm not myself anymore. I feel lost, and it's hard to accept this. I'm used to helping others and…" The phone rang, and her secretary's voice was heard through the phone.

"Dr. Givins, your husband, would like to speak with you on line one."

"Excuse me, Samone, but I have to take this call."

While she was on the phone, I began to think, *"I can't believe this; I'm going to have to get off this medication by myself and believe me, I have already tried; it's hard. I feel drained and without energy. My stomach feels upset and I feel as if I need to vomit. It's a horrible feeling and it seems that will be the only way I get off it."*

"Yes, Dear…I know. Well, Sweetie, I'm in the middle of… well if you don't care, then I don't care."

I'm no dummy; she was really trying to pretend with her voice that she was having a pleasant conversation when she wasn't. It was written all over her face. Besides that, I could hear her husband screaming at her from the other end. She hung up the phone and cleared her throat.

"I apologize for that, Ms. Grey. You may finish what you were saying." The phone rang again.

"Dr. Givins, your husband is…" Before her secretary finished speaking, Dr. Givins told her not to send through any more calls for the morning.

"As you wish, Dr. Givins."

"Thanks, Gladys."

"So, you are very important to your husband, huh?"

She looked at me with piercing eyes that said, "How dare you ask me a question about my personal life. Excuse me, what do you mean by that, Samone?"

"Oh, I just admire a woman who has a husband that calls her at her job and yells at her because she is in a better career arena than he is, that's all."

With the confidence that my words would melt the very thin and slippery ice-cold conversation, I gleamed for the response, and what do you know, it worked. Smiling and exhaling, she thanked me for the witty sarcasm.

"No problem, Dr. Givens."

"Now, what were you saying?" She pulled out my folder and began to write something.

"Oh, uh…well, I was basically trying to change your mind about not helping me."

"But, I am helping you, Samone. Frankly, you need those prescriptions if they are not harming you physically. You will be able to have a handle on those racing thoughts, and besides that, they do help you sleep, right?" She was right again; in fact, that's all I wanted to do.

With reluctance, I answered, "Yes."

"Is there anything on your mind that bothers you right now, and if so, would you like to talk about it?"

I thought about my job and the stress that came with it. I was very good at keeping things to myself, but that would defeat the purpose of seeing a shrink. So, I let all my problems out dealing with my job.

I told her about the woman who kept the place up and running. Now, I must admit, the woman does her job extremely well, but she keeps up a lot of drama. The whole building knows about this obnoxious woman. I try to keep a sane head around her, but sometimes I just want to scream at the top of my lungs at her. She walks around, griping at this person and that person about what job they have done incorrectly. Try to imagine a bulldog lurking in the office, sniffing out something that is trouble; that is her. I continued to wonder why she is still employed, but an answer hasn't been given. She makes everyone have headaches, and a co-worker of mine said she had a heart attack because of her. To me, that is an extreme need to get rid of someone. But, that is not how the corporate world works. The bosses and supervisors keep whoever helps them out the most, regardless of the treatment they give to others.

It felt good to release my worries to someone who was trained on stress and other mental issues. I explained to her how I had an episode due to the stress I received from this woman.

I was sitting at my desk, and it hit me. I went into a trance that left me staring at the computer screen, trying to remember what to do next. I remember thinking I was contacting the dead and that they were using my body as their very own. Sounds creepy, huh? Well, try living it. I was so out of it, but I was able to snap back, somehow. It was a scary experience for me, one I would not wish upon anyone to experience. After the episode was over, I gathered my sane thoughts together and began to work once again. I explained all of this to her without feeling embarrassed or ashamed, and she made me feel so comfortable.

"Samone, what kind of work do you do?"

"I work for the State of Texas as an Administrative Assistant."

"Do you like your job?"

"I love my job; I love what I do, but if things don't get better with that woman, I'm going to have to quit. I know that stress can kill you, and that woman is stressing me out. How can I handle the stress I receive from this woman?"

"Well, Samone, you are going to have to find a way to release your thoughts and act out your emotions in a positive, but yet, firm way." I guess she could tell I was already trying to think of a way right then and there from my facial expression.

"Samone, you don't have to do it right now. I have noticed from your conversations that you tend to change it quickly to explain something else. Try to slowly explain your point of view of a subject before you move on to the next subject."

"Dr. Givins, I can't help it; that's just how my mind moves. I think people should just try to keep up." She let out a small laugh of sarcasm.

"Ms. Grey, please give thought to what you are going to say before you say it. It helps."

"Dr. Givins, I don't mean to be rude, but my thoughts are the problem here. You are the doctor, so you should know what symptoms I am experiencing."

"Well, honestly, Samone, your diagnosis can't be totally correct because bipolar generally affects the person's mood swing instead of the thoughts, but sometimes they go hand in hand. Like, in your case."

I sat in this wonderful, comfortable, exquisite chair and pondered on what she just told me. Could Dr. Lim be incorrect about me being bipolar? If so, what am I?

"Well, could you tell me the correct diagnoses?"

"Well, Samone, that depends on a number of things, but it seems to me that you have a disorder called Schizoaffective Disorder Bipolar Type."

"Schizo…who?"

"Schizoaffective Disorder Bipolar Type."

"Dr. Givins, you are really worth your money if you can just tell by one conversation and meeting with me that I am something totally different than my last diagnosis. I mean, that is something I have never heard of, and you just want me to accept it. What does it mean?"

"Ms. Grey, I have been doing this job for a good while now, and I just shared something with you that I generally wouldn't. If you were completely bipolar, you wouldn't be experiencing things as you did at your job. That is just not bipolar symptoms, but to answer your question, schizoaffective disorder is being in between schizophrenic and bipolar. The person would have symptoms of both, and Ms. Grey, you have the symptoms of both. I also think that your medicine may be too strong, which is your reason for wanting to discontinue. Therefore, you should obtain a new prescription from me. I will give it to you before you leave." I had so many questions running through my mind, but I only asked her one.

"What are the symptoms of schizophrenia?"

"I have some information available for patients who don't have a complete understanding of what their diagnosis is." She bent over and opened her file cabinet and pulled out a packet with an overview of a Schizoaffective Disorder Bipolar Type.

"Here you go, Samone; I hope it gives you the information you are seeking, and if not, pick up the phone and give me a call."

She looked at her watch, and so did I. It had almost been an hour, and we didn't realize it; well, maybe I didn't. She began to fill out my prescription while I stood waiting. When she was finished, she handed it to me with a nice warm smile.

"Ok, Ms. Grey, I need you to see the secretarial desk to schedule another appointment, three weeks from today. Be sure to call if you have any problems with the medication. Take one pill at night, at bedtime."

"Okay, Thanks, Dr. Givins."

She stood and we shook hands, then I exited the door. I left that office feeling superior; noticing that feeling made me think that she's a really good doctor.

On the bus ride home, it was packed with people. Some were sitting, others were stooping, and there were people in my predicament who was standing. I thought about trying to read that packet, but I decided not to because of all the people around me. I didn't want anyone to suspect anything. So, I just looked out the window and awaited my arrival to my stop. There was a commotion going on at the front of the bus.

"Look, I just want you to shut your kids up, that's all. Could you do that?" It was a man's voice overpowering the young mother, who was trying to state her case.

"Could you just mind your own business and shut up?"

The children must have hated seeing their mother arguing because they started crying even more. I tried to imagine myself with three children at the age of 26; I couldn't. It must be hard trying to lug children around to take care of business for home. The young woman was professionally dressed; she looked as if she had been on a job interview. Her hair was in a nicely done French roll with wavy young curls in front. She had high cheekbones and full lips with pink lip gloss on them. Her skin matched the color of cinnamon brown with very few blemishes. The auburn color skirt suit matched perfectly with her skin. She was a nice looking lady.

The man had on brown looking slacks with a tan dress shirt. His shoes were shiny and delightful to look at. He looked to be in his early 30s. Like the young woman, he was good looking as well. He just had an awful attitude, which made him ugly.

They calmed down, and so did the children. People can really make a scene when they want to. I don't understand why they both had to get loud over the noise that the children made.

The bus finally made its way to the street of my apartment complex. As I was heading towards my apartment, something started to vibrate in my bag. Hurriedly, I opened my bag and reached for my cell phone.

"Hi, Mama. How are you doing?"

"I'm doing good, Baby; I'm making it."

"That's good to hear."

"How did your appointment go?"

"Oh, it went well, although she gave me another diagnosis."

"Oh really, what was it or is it?"

"Yeah, she called it a schizoaffective disorder."

"What is that?"

"I don't know just yet, but she gave me a packet to read for information."

"Well, that's good. You know your boyfriend is in jail, right?" I stopped at my last step to climb.

"Whhaat? What is he in jail for? What did he do this time?"

"Oh, don't act dumb Samone, you know he is still selling that crack, weed, marijuana, whatever it's called."

"Mama, I know what he told me he was going to stop doing. I can't believe this; he keeps lying to me. How did you find out anyway?"

"Your sister called and told me. Baby, you really need to let him go. He is no good for you, Samone. Listen to your Mama, I know."

I tried to gather my thoughts, for I felt them beginning to race again. I really need to get that medicine, and I hope it works well enough.

"Mama, I know what I need to do, but I love him. How do I give up love like that?"

"Samone, you know what you need to do. He has been in your pockets for money a lot lately. Look at what he is doing to you. That's all you really need to do is see his faults."

"Mama, everybody's in my pockets nowadays." There was silence for about half a minute. I had just loaned her some money two days ago.

"I know you are not referring to me, are you? Because you know I'm going to pay you back your money."

"Mama, I'm frustrated right now. No, I'm not talking about you." I lied. I could tell I made my mother upset, and she decided to get off the phone with me.

"Alright, Mama, I'll talk to you later, and thanks for the bad news."

I know Joshua will call me to bail him out of jail, but I'm not. This is his second time going to jail for drugs. Why won't he learn? I opened the door to my apartment while dialing my sister's number.

"Hello. How did you find out Joshua is in jail before me?"

"Because he told me."

"How? He's in jail."

"Samone, come on now; you know he must have called me then."

"Don't get smart with me Dedra. I just asked a question." For some reason, she was really nasty to me and I hadn't done anything.

"First of all, why are you so nasty with me, and I haven't done anything to you?"

"Samone, Girl, you need to just calm down because I'm not even trippin'. Your boyfriend called me with his bad news." I calmed down because she had calmed down. Her voice was at a better tone, a level I could handle.

"Did he tell you why he called you and not me?"

"He told me that he knew you would be upset. So, he called me to call you."

"But Dedra, you called Mama first and whoever else."

"Don't worry. Mama is the only person I told. I don't know who she may have told, though. I'm sorry for telling Mama. I told her to let me tell you first, but obviously that went into one ear and out the other. I don't know why Mama couldn't wait for me to tell you."

"I know why, because she can't stand Joshua."

"Sis, you do need to let him go, though."

"I know and I will."

"You said that before."

"I know, but I mean it this time." My house phone rang.

"Girl, that must be him; let me call you back."

"Ok, bye."

"Bye."

I answered my phone, "Hello."

You have an incoming call from... (I heard his deep voice say Joshua) would you like to accept the call? I replied, "yes."

"Hello."

"Hey Baby, I'm sorry, for I already know what you are going to say."

"Make it quick Joshua. I have no tolerance for this anymore."

"Baby, I'm sorry. You are the only person I have. Can you come and bail me out?" I was a good woman to my man, but a huge light was beginning to shine and let me know that this was no man but a boy.

"Baby, I love you, but I can't. You are just going to have to do your time. Besides, I don't have enough money to cover your bail."

"Baby." A woman's voice came over the phone to announce the minutes that passed/two minutes passed.

"It won't cost that much because I only had weed on me. Everybody knows that you only have a minimum that you have to come up with. So, can I depend on you this last time?" I was going to be strong this time, no matter what.

"I mean it Joshua, this better be your last time, but you are gonna' have to call me when you get out on your own." I hung up the phone.

I began to cry because I felt I had just done the most horrible thing in the world. I grabbed my keys and headed to the nearby Walgreens to put my new prescription in. They told me it would be at least an hour before they could fill it. Therefore, I decided to pick it up the next day. As I was leaving the store, I ran into an old friend. He has always had the biggest crush on me ever since I can remember.

"Hey Charles, what's up."

"Nuttin' much just chillin'. Up in this store trying to find me a woman." He smiled as to say he was just kidding, "whatchu' doin' up in here?" I must have been a fool to have dated this nut for a short time. I hated the way he spoke. He did not know about my condition, so I decided to keep it that way.

"Oh, I came in here to get some cleaning products."

"Oh, for real. Why don't chu' have no bags den'?"

"Because I decided not to get them at the last minute."

I lied to him because I didn't want him to find out the real reason for being at Walgreens. It must be his looks that always attracted me to this man because he still looks the same. Damn good, real good… good enough to eat. I began to look him over but stopped because of my thoughts of Joshua, work, and my condition.

"Are you a'ight Samone? I love the way you make me moan." He started chuckling at his own inside joke. He used to always say that after we had sex.

"Yeah, I'm alright; just a little tired."

"You kno' I can take care of you, right?"

I looked at him and knew that he was being honest. Charles had never cheated on me when we dated. He smoked, drank, and used incorrect grammar, which turned me off. If he would only change those details about himself, he may be a perfect match for me, but we will remain friends until then.

"You need a ride home?" At first, I wasn't going to take him up on his offer, but then I realized I had quite a long walk to make.

"Yeah, I would."

"Kewl, come on."

He led me out of the store and guided me to his silver 2004 Impala. Charles opened my door for me and I slid in. Yeah, Charles is a real gentleman, but yet he has thuggish ways. He jumped in the car and started the motor. Of course, he had the music blaring from his speakers. Actually, it was someone I liked. Charles pulled on Riverside and headed in my direction.

"Ok, Samone, why did you break up wit' me? I mean, I treated you good, and I gotta tell you, I still love you." I looked at him, but his eyes were on the road.

"Charles, I told you why we couldn't work. You are too gangsta for me."

"Mone, I can't help the way I am. It's just who I am."

"And I understand that; you must respect my decision now."

"You are sump tin' else Mone. You would rather let me go and put up wit' that sorry excuse of a brother. You must don't know he in jail and you talking about me being gangsta… this man sells for a living. You know those types of men have guns and shit, and you have the nerve to complain about me. I got you, Samone, I understand." I got quiet, which I usually don't do since I always have a remark. My eyes were on the road this time.

"Why you so quiet? What? You don't think I keep up with you and what goes on with you?" While I was turning to face him, he parked the car. I inhaled a deep breath, not knowing what to say to what he had found out.

"How did you find out about Joshua?"

"Word git' around the street pretty fas.' Besides, you know yo' man sell, and you know I be lookin' for something to smoke."

"You really do need to quit smoking that stuff." I was embarrassed that everyone knew about Joshua before I did and I was his woman.

"Don't turn the story around on me. You still haven't answered my question."

"Do you want the honest truth?"

We were both facing each other. With the gas prices continually rising, I thought he would want to turn his air off, but it was too hot for that. Texas is custom to being hot.

"Why don't we finish dis' conversation inside yo' apartment, and yes, I want you to be honest. I never want you to lie to me."

"Naww, we can finish it right here. It won't take long. The truth is, Charles, I am very attracted to you, but you smoke, drink, and use slang to the point that sometimes I don't know what you are saying."

I looked away, but he turned my face back to him and landed a nice big kiss on me. I wasn't expecting that, so I reacted very shocked. He smiled and showed his dimples.

"You like that kind of stuff, don't you? I remember you telling me you like to be caught off guard when it comes to kisses."

Racing thoughts began to reappear. Charles acts as if nothing I said bothered him. What was wrong with the man? Does he really care for me? Maybe he does; I just don't know how to handle it. He landed another one, and this time I kissed back. His lips were soft and enjoyable, but I had to stop myself, though, because of Joshua. I couldn't stop thinking about him during the whole 10-second kiss. I pulled away from him; he gave me a dumbfounded look. He then tried to lean in for a third, but I pushed him back into his seat.

"Look, we got to stop this. We can't allow ourselves to give in into emotions that are not there."

"So, what do you mean? You sayin' you don't ever want to be with me again? Because if that's the case, why did you kiss back? I think you still want me, but you are mixed up with that fool of a man."

"Umm, wait a minute…isn't he that same fool that gives you what you want?"

"What? Why you taking up for 'em? He out there selling dangerous drugs, and you are condoning it."

"Hold up, wait a minute. I never said I agree with what he is doing. I'm just trying to bring to your attention of how you look as well. You are no angle, so don't try to act like one." There was silence in the car for about three minutes. Both of us were very heated.

"Well, look, Charles, I'm not going to sit here and pretend that all the feelings I had for you are totally gone; they are still there. It's just it's just… well the fact of the matter is that Joshua is still around. Therefore, I'm in no need for another relationship." Charles just stared straight through me as I told him my thoughts. He looked at me as if he didn't hear a word I said.

"Look, Samone, I'm going to give you time to make a decision. I know you don't wanna' let me go completely. You still need some Charles in your life." I looked at him with timid eyes, which told him my thoughts.

"I know you think you don't need me right now, Samone but you do, and I'm gonna have you as my woman."

Now he made me mad; he didn't listen to a word I just said. Now don't get me wrong, I liked his boldness and persistence, but man, he needed to calm down a little. I got out of the car and bent down so that I could see within the window.

"Charles, I will definitely give you a call when I'm ready for another relationship."

"Mone, don't be lying, tell the truth. Are you gonna call me?"

"Yes, Charles, I will give you a call. Now please leave before my man pulls up."

"He gotta git' out of jail first to do dat." The car began to roll back slowly, with him yelling things out of the car.

"I bet he can't love you like I can! Bet he can't!"

I was beginning to get embarrassed because I was pretty sure people could hear what he said to me. But inside, I felt good to have a man yelling things that many women would dream for a man to say. Trust me when I say that I believed in Charles's words that he said to me. I don't know why I did, but I did. Then something hit me; Charles knows how to use correct English, for he proved it by the way he was speaking to me.

Dimples were gone and he left me standing there looking after his car. Realizing that he was gone, I walked to my apartment and found something to eat. The 9 o'clock news would be on shortly, so I decided to fix something quick to eat. I made spaghetti and cheese with my famous garlic bread. Maybe I should have invited Charles in; it would have been promising. He would have told some jokes and made me laugh. I wonder if he would be willing to turn around and swing back by. I was scrolling through my cell phone when I thought it would be best to wait. Charles is just too demanding right now and besides, he probably would try to have sex with me. He is just the type that would do something like, try to give me a message and give me unnecessary kisses like he did in the car. He knows I get a thrill off that kind of thing and he'll used it to his advantage. Just thinking about that, I quickly changed my mind.

I sat down to eat dinner alone at my dinette set. The kitchen area of my apartment is open and spacious. The dinette table faced towards the living room so that I was able to see the television. I grabbed the remote and pushed the power button. As I sat down in my chair, I heard the anchorwoman, Janice Calbright, say, "Good evening, and thank you for joining us for the 9 o'clock news. This evening we are going to cover stories dealing with drugs in our communities, and here with me is Michael Brock to help discuss the issues that we are facing, Michael."

"Good evening, our first story takes place in Houston…" Just as I was getting into the news, the phone rang.

I thought to myself, *"This had better be an important call, for whomever, it was going make me miss the news."*

I picked up the phone and heard an imitating voice say, "I know what you are doing and I know what you did last summer."

I giggled and said, "And I know who you are, Michelle."

She pretended not to hear me and replied, "You are watching T.V. right now; I can see you through the window."

I got up from the chair and checked the window to see if she was really there. When I saw her thick figure standing in the window where she began to laugh. I opened the front door and she stepped in. We hugged each other; she then headed towards the kitchen.

"I came at perfect timing, didn't I?"

"I guess you did; I was wondering who was going to show up and help me eat up my food."

"Aww, Girl, you know I will be thrilled to do the job." She fixed herself a plate and made her way to the table.

"So, what do you know?"

"Well, what I know is you already know that my man is in jail; tell me if you don't know."

Michelle let out her screeching little laugh and said, "But of course I know, because you know that your man and my man are best friends."

"So when did Tyrone tell you?"

"He told me earlier today." She and I both put food in our mouths and began to chew; I swallowed first.

"Did he try to call you yet?"

"Eww, don't talk with your mouth full of food; that's disgusting," I said.

She showed me her tongue covered with food and said, "Aww, don't act like you never did it."

"You are nasty Michelle; I want you to know that."

"I know I am and my man do too."

"Aww, here we go. So, how are you and Mr. Green doing?"

"We are doing good. In fact, that's why I came over here to ask you something. But before I do, you have to answer my question first. Samone, what in the hell made you hang up on the man? Don't you know he has the most pay in all of Texas when it comes to a man selling drugs? I know he is filthy rich."

"Well, why did he ask me to bail him out, if he's so rich?"

"I don't know. Maybe, he was just testing you to see if you would. You know, men have their little games they play just like we do." I studied her while I was in deep thought and realized that she could be right.

"Joshua knows better than to play games with me. I tell him all the time that I need him to be straight forward and honest with me, and he has been as far as I'm concerned. He tells me all about his drug deals, parties, ex women, friends, and etc."

"That's good; he is honest about some things, but know that men keep a lot of things secret. Trust me Samone, I know." She sounded as if she was holding something back.

"Do you know something that I don't, Michelle?"

"Naw Girl, what are you talking about? I'm just saying, all men keep secrets just like women," she said then changed the subject real quick by asking me, "have you told him about Charles yet?" I sometimes hate that I even told her about Charles. Now, she holds it over my head like she wants to tell him herself.

"Yeah, I told him…in so many words."

"Whateva' you know you didn't tell him. I don't know why you are trying to front like you have."

"Because Joshua knows Charles and if he finds out that I had a relationship with him…God only knows what he would do. I will tell him one day soon."

"Well, YOUR secret is safe with me. I won't tell him or Ty."

"Now you know if you tell Ty, that's just like telling Joshua himself, so don't even bring Ty in this."

"You my girl, I wouldn't do that to you. I'll let you tell Joshua on your own time." We finished dinner and headed towards the living room. She stretched out on my couch that was made for two and exhaled.

"Ahh, I could just fall asleep right here. I don't know where you found these couches, but they are so comfortable. It's like sitting on soft feathers."

My living room consisted of two brown leather couches, one state of the art brown/red lazy boy chair, and a thirty-two-inch television set. I had the television in a nice oak wood entertainment center. The end tables and center table match perfectly with the entertainment center, for they were the same color. Underneath the center table laid a nice expensive rug with red, brown, and tan colors. The tan in the rug brings out the red in the African masks I have on the walls. I must say I have nice taste; my living room always gets compliments from visitors.

"Well, just go on to sleep. You already made me miss your sister tonight."

"Aww, she will be on tomorrow; she really takes that job to her head, you know."

"She is supposed to; she is on the news where thousands of people look at her every night. Maybe you should think about covering for her when she becomes ill. Y'all look so much alike."

I knew she was going to go off on me by saying that. Michelle hated being compared or thought of as being like her sister, Janice Carlbright. She didn't say one thing which surprised the hell out of me.

"Oh yeah, Michelle, what were you going to ask me?"

She quickly sat up with a goofy smile on her face and said, "Would you be my maid of honor?"

At first, I didn't know what to say because this was an extremely important decision that she obviously made. She had only been dating Tyrone for six months and now she's getting married.

"Wuuhh...Tyrone Green asked you to marry him?"

She shook her head yes vigorously, "Yeah, he asked me yesterday; I can't believe it. I'm going to get married." Deep inside, I was disappointed for her because of Tyrone's job profession, but I played it off and pretended to be happy for her.

"Girl, I'm so excited for you." She could tell I was lying, by the way I said it.

"Samone, you really are ruining my mood here; you are supposed to be happy for me, not faking like you are. You should know me better than that. I can suspect when something is wrong with you." I sat across from her on my couch with three seats, but I moved to sit right next to her.

"What were you thinking about when you agreed to marry him? I mean, the dude is a drug dealer and he isn't a small timer either."

"Wow, that's how you feel about my decision, you of all people. Don't act so innocent your man is the top-dog on the chain. Tyrone answers to him. I know he sells drugs, but I love him with all of me. And to tell you the truth, I know he loves me. So that's why we both agreed to get married. I can't believe you are so jealous." She stood up and started pacing the floor.

"Hold on, wait one minute." I put my index finger up and started shaking it to say no.

"I am not jealous of nobody. If I really wanted to get married, I would have been already. Don't ever think I haven't been asked before because I have and it was recently, for that matter." I tried to calm down, for Michelle was making me very vexed. She stood there looking at me like I was a stranger she did not know.

"Michelle, marriage is a huge commitment that both of you may still be too young for. You are only 19-years-old and he is 21; well, he may be ready, but I seriously doubt it."

"See, this is the thing Samone," she said very angrily, "I know my age and I know what I want. I know how to commit and I know how to love. Those are all the things you need first to be seriously thinking about marriage. Someone may have asked you a long time ago to marry them, but you are so stubborn with just letting go and letting someone love you that you are alone and hurting. You would be surprised as to what a man would do for you if you would give him your all."

I told Michelle about all the details of my relationships except one. There was one man that I gave my all to and he broke my heart in half. I let her continue on with her explanation with anger.

"Samone, I hope you are listening to me when I say that Joshua and Ty are going to be just fine. Joshua may be in jail, but trust me, he has money to spare. Ty told me that he was working on getting his bail today and that he should be out by tomorrow morning. I know I might sound a little angry, but I'm just frustrated by how you are looking at my situation." She got quiet and sat down in the lazy boy.

"Chelle, I just want you to know that I respect you and your decisions. I was only concerned about your wellbeing. Your heart holds all your emotions in it and I don't want to see it get broken in half. You are a very sweet person and you deserve better, just like I do. The men that we have are drug dealers and that's no good. How does it make us look to other people? You know they got to wonder, what kind of woman we are that would date such men." It was no getting through to her, for she exhaled with an irritating noise. That's when I knew she was really into the game with Tyrone.

"So, are you going to be in my wedding or what?"

"Of course, I am."

"Good. Well, I'm fixin' to head on out it's getting late and Tyrone is probably looking for me."

She never left on a note like that. She was always willing to spend a night and Ty hardly ever said anything about it. That's how I knew she was really upset with me. She may seem calm, but deep inside, she was pissed off.

"Alright, if that's what you want to do."

"Yeeaah, I'm gonna head on home tonight." She grabbed her keys and headed towards the door.

"Thanks for dinner and I will talk with you tomorrow."

"Alright, you be safe driving, ok."

"Ok, bye."

"Bye."

I closed the door behind her and went to run my bathwater. I was pretty tense after the heated conversation. So I knew that a bath with music and candles would be an excellent relaxing method for me.

CHAPTER TWO

Sade was playing through the speakers as I slid into the tub of nice hot water. Bubbles were everywhere and they seemed to add on to the relaxing atmosphere that I had set up. I inhaled the aroma and held it before I exhaled. I don't know why, but baths always calm me down mentally and physically.

"This is No Ordinary Love.. No Ordinary Love," I sang along.

I was grooving and feeling somewhat better when the phone rang. I wondered who it could be since it was after eleven. I didn't bother to answer it because of my bath. So, I sat there and just let the phone ring. It rang about five times before the person hung up and tried again.

After about 30 minutes, the water began to chill and I took that as my sign for getting out. I stepped out the tub and dried myself off with one of those big huge beach towels. I made sure I was completely dry before I rubbed my lotion on. People always compliment me on my skin and they always asked me my secret. I never told them that all they had to do is make sure their skin is completely dry before applying lotion. It leaves the skin very soft and at a glow. I slipped into my "happy" pajamas. My pajamas reminded me of myself; they were covered with red hearts and yellow smiley faces. I let the water out, washed my face, brushed my teeth, and now, I was ready for bed. Before I slid into my bed, I checked the caller ID to see who it was that called. The number looked familiar, but I couldn't recall who it belongs to. Laying down, I turned off the lights and continued the play of Sade. I laid there thinking about the conversation with Michelle. I knew she was going to tell Ty that could have been him trying to call me, but I didn't give it any second thought. I could feel myself drifting off to sleep, but my mind was not willing.

The next thing I knew, I felt a force of wind or better known as a spirit, hoover over me like I was its soul to partake. It embarked my mind and I heard a voice called out my name.

"Samone." I remember thinking is this for real or is my mind playing tricks on me.

The spirit called out my name a second time, "Samone!"

"Here I am, what do you want?" I asked, horrified.

"Samone, do you know who I am?"

I shook my head to recover my saneness, but it didn't work for the spirit just kept repeating the same question repeatedly. I tried to get from my bed, but I couldn't move. My head started to shake on its own and that really freaked me out because I was logically coherent, but I couldn't stop what was going on. My life, health, and most of all, my mind all blinked within seconds before me. I was helpless; I couldn't do anything, but just wait until it ended. The whole ordeal lasted for about two minutes, but it felt like 10 to me.

Being able to move again, I looked at the clock and the red digital light read 11:45. I proceeded to move from my bed and went into the bathroom. I opened the medicine cabinet and swallowed my old prescription. I thought I would be able to go one day without taking my meds, but I obviously can't. I didn't realize how screwed up my mind was until now. I mean, I first noticed the problem in 2004 when I was employed at a bank. I remember having thoughts that told me to quit my job and be employed with another within days. I also remember writing notes of this glorious wedding I was supposed to have, the people that would be there, and the location of where it would be. At first, I thought God spoke to me through my mind and not my heart, but it ended up not being the case. Not receiving any medical attention then has left my mind to suffer somewhat. I didn't get diagnosed until 2005, which to me is a long time to be suffering from a mental disorder and not even know it. There are still things I don't know about myself now. I don't understand delusions in the mind.

Doctors continually ask me if I suffer from suicidal thoughts, hear any voices or if I have any hallucinations. I tell them no each time because I don't really want to feel insecure, but the fact of the matter is, I do. The next doctor's visit, I will definitely tell the truth.

After taking my old prescription, I began to feel somewhat better. I called my mother and explained everything that happened.

"Mama, I swear someone or something called out my name. It was so real to be false."

"Baby, now you know you suffer from those things. Did you take your medicine?"

"I just took it 30 minutes ago before I called you. I'm starting to feel it now."

"Do you need someone to come over and spend the night with you? You sound so scared."

"I really do want someone to come over, but I don't expect anyone to get out of bed and come over here. Besides, this medicine is making me sleepy, so I will probably be alright."

"Are you sure, because I will come over if you want?"

"Mama I'm sure, it's just good to hear someone's voice that is really real."

"How does your head feel right now? Does it hurt?"

"Yeah, it hurts a little bit, but I can handle it. Thanks for talking with me Mama; maybe I just needed to hear someone's voice."

"You are welcome, Baby. Do you think you are going to make it to work tomorrow?"

"No, not after what happened. I'm going to take a couple of days off."

"Good. Just try not to lose your job this time. You have a good job Samone, so try to keep it."

"I'm working on not losing my job. Ma don't worry about it, I got it covered." My mother comforted me with more words before she hung up and when she did, I slept like a baby.

The next morning, I called in. My supervisor, Brenda Jackson was concerned; she kept pressuring me to give details as to why I couldn't make it in. I told her about my headache and not being able to stay focused. Then she agreed to an off period of two days.

Now that I had two days to refocus, I was going to use it to the fullest. I needed to figure out what to do with Joshua, Charles, and myself. I needed short term goals to follow through for me. I got up to brush my teeth and wash my face when I suddenly heard the doorbell ring. Chills went down my back for I had a feeling it was Joshua. No one else that I knew would show up at my apartment at 6:30 in the morning but him and it made me nervous. I gathered my composure and went to open the door.

"Who is it?" I asked through the door.

"Open the door and see." I knew that voice; I was right it was Joshua.

I hesitated before opening the door. I didn't know what to expect from him since I hung up the phone on him.

He strode through my door with roses in his hand. He handed the flowers to me and then leaned in for a kiss. I accepted the roses, but I didn't accept his invitation for a kiss. He looked at me dumbfounded and tried again. I rejected him a second time.

"What's with you, Samone? You haven't seen me in two weeks and you are acting shady." He began to look around my apartment for I guess, some other man. I stood there looking bewildered because he had the audacity to do such a thing.

While he was still looking around, I yelled out in anger, "You will not find anyone here! I don't know why you are looking around in my apartment the way you are!" I followed him into my bedroom to see exactly what he had found, for he stayed in there longer than he did any other room.

"Come here; I want to talk with you."

He was sitting on my bed with his head in his hands. I was angry and annoyed. I really didn't feel like talking to him, but I went over anyway. I decided to let him do all the talking.

"I want you to know that you hurt me when you hung up on me. I just knew you were with someone else. Why did you do such a thing? I feel as if I can't trust you anymore." I looked in his teddy bear brown eyes and began to state my case.

"First of all..."

"Wait a minute, Samone, you are already starting your explanation off wrong. Just calm down and talk to me without an attitude."

"Don't come in here telling me what to do in my own place. If I want to start off like I was, then let me do so. First of all, you don't know how much you have hurt me with your continuous lying. You said you were going to stop selling and you have not. Then you turn around and want me to bail you out of jail. I don't understand you Joshua. You expect so much from people and you don't give back. You need to realize that I want different things now. At first, it was alright with you dealing drugs; I didn't understand what I was really getting myself into. Now that I know, maann I don't want to be a part of it anymore." The whole time I was speaking, he looked at me in my eyes as if he were searching for me to lie to him.

When he didn't find anything, he said, "Look, I understand you are upset about the whole drug situation of mine. And you are wrong; I never told you a lie. I told you I was going to quit, but I never told you when. I need to find a job that will accept me first. Just about everyone in Texas knows about me. I love you, Samone, I always have and will. You just need to be patient and give me time to get myself together. I didn't pay off judges and lawyers this week for me to come here and get treated this way. I came here for love from my woman. You are still my woman, right? Don't tell me no lie either; if you are seeing someone else, then let me know right now." I could see it in his handsome face that he was being sincere or at least I thought he was.

"I don't have anyone else; I barely can keep up with you."

He let out a laugh, "That's why I love you so much; you always know how to make me laugh even when I don't want to." I was sitting close enough to him where he could kiss me on the forehead.

"I didn't mean that to be funny. You are a handful Joshua and I hope you know that."

"I know, and you are too. It's a wonder you don't have another man on the side."

"Why, are you suggesting it? Do you think I should?"

He scratched his head and said, "Do you want another man?" I hated it when he answered a question with a question; only I could do that.

"No, I don't want another man. I just want one man to get his shit together and act right." He looked at me with shock in his eyes.

"We are using profanity now?" I hardly ever used profanity; I only used it when I was angry.

I shied with a smile and said, "Umm… oops." He let out another laugh.

"You know what Samone?"

"What?"

"You are very cute when you are upset. It makes me want you."

I knew I wasn't supposed to be enjoying his company right now, but I was. We were supposed to be breaking up, but we weren't; we were making up. I can't understand myself sometimes, I make plans, but I don't follow through with them.

I played dumb and replied, "Want me how?"

Joshua looked at me with desirable eyes and said, "How do you think?"

I thought to myself, *"There he go again, answering my question with a question."* But I knew exactly what he wanted to do. He got down between my legs on his knees and looked up to my face.

"I just want you to know that I sincerely apologize for not being upfront with you about my plans of quitting the dope game. I love you and I don't want to see another brother with you. So, promise me you will be patient with me."

"Look, I love you too, Joshua, but it's hard knowing what you do can affect me somehow. What if someone decided they wanted to take your position and come for me?"

"They won't come after you, I promise. Can you make a promise to me? Can you wait for me to get my shit together?"

"I can't promise that. I mean, I can promise that I won't date anyone else for a good while if we should break up."

All the while that I was saying my speech, my thoughts were: *dump him, let him go, you know what people are going to think. You need to be by yourself for a while, come on Samone, you can do it.*

I ignored my personal thoughts and finished my speech, "The way you make your living really scares me Joshua and I don't know how much longer I can put up with it." He got up from the floor, grabbed me close, and shushed me like I was some kind of child.

"Don't worry about me Samone, I know how to work the system. Just trust me; everything will work out fine. You have to just give it time." I didn't say anything; I just let him hold me in his arms and inhaled his scent. He gently put my head in his hands, then he began to stroke my micro braids.

"You are so beautiful, never forget that Samone no matter what."

Looking within his teddy bear, brown eyes made me realize how handsome he is. His long neck makes him look twice his height which in actuality is 6'1; his body consisted of impeccable muscles and flawless weight. His dark chocolate skin color drove me nuts; I just loved it. He has a nice set of white teeth that shines so bright that you would think you were staring at light. Being pretty hip, Joshua inclined to be like most, preceding the goatee and thin hairline upon the jawbone. He could go for a model out of a magazine. His high cheekbones made his smile out of this world. He doesn't own any dimples, but his smile is worth the while to just stare at.

Joshua's pride and joy is his hair. I never knew a man that pays such attention and detail to his hair the way he did. He didn't allow many to touch his hair either. To tell you the truth, I only know of one woman who braids his hair and she is well paid for it too. He usually keeps it braided most of the time. He says it's much easier for his everyday life. Joshua has a way that he speaks to me that drive shivers up and down my back. His voice is rich, deep, and admirable for some. At times when I have a hard day, he can just come in and soothe my problems away with his cool, calm, and suave ways. I really love that about him. He is persistent, straight forward, and honest as they come. The only thing that I regret about him is his profession. I love the man and there is no doubt in my mind that I do. I just want him to find a 9 to 5.

"One day Samone when I get myself together, I want you to be the mother of my children. I want you to have everything. It is my desire that you be mine forever." It was after 7 a.m., and this man was saying such loving words in my ears. I never thought I would have a man in my life that would say such darling things. Now that he was in my life, I didn't know how to react.

"I love you Joshua Eugene Franks, I really do."

After I had said that, I leaned in and kissed him. It was such an intense moment; I could feel the fire rising between us. It had been a whole month since I have had sex. He started backing me up towards the bed while kissing me. He landed on top of me when we made it to the bed. The kisses began to become deeper and faster. I felt his nature rise and I was on fire. His hand was on my left breast; he started squeezing it with gentle force; I moaned with delight. My lips were on his neck, kissing and licking with such ease that he let out a moan.

"Samone, I missed you," he whispered in my ear.

"I've missed you too."

He then took me to a place where I haven't been in a month, a place where I forgot about all my problems and misfortunes. For some reason, it was the best sex we had since we have been together. Maybe it was because it was "makeup" sex, I don't know, but it was brilliant.

After we were finished, I said, "You really were great Joshua. You totally satisfied my needs on this beautiful morning."

"So, the morning is beautiful to you now, huh…since you got a piece of me? I'm glad I could be of assistance to you."

Smiling, I said, "Hopefully, it was good for you too."

He looked at me with amazement then he replied, "Oooo Weee! It was the best we have had in a good while."

"I know, tell me about it."

We entered into the bathroom to relieve ourselves from the aroma that had accumulated upon our bodies. The shower was nice and spicy, for we went at it again while showering. I tell you the truth when I say; I just couldn't keep my hands off of him. I felt on top of the world and he helps me get there. Feeling fresh and clean, I headed toward the kitchen to stir us up some breakfast. I was feeling really good, so I decided to make the works. I left Joshua in the bathroom, but he soon appeared.

"So, Ms. Lady what are you cooking me for breakfast?"

Smiling at him, I said, "I'm making pancakes, grits, turkey bacon, eggs, and toast. Do you think that will satisfy your appetite?"

He was standing behind me, he kissed me on the neck, and he whispered in my ear, "I don't know, maybe?"

Giggling, I said, "Com' on now, let's eat breakfast first before we do that again. You are wearing me out."

He walked to the kitchen table and grabbed an old newspaper and began to read; while reading, he said, "See, Samone I told you that you wouldn't be able to handle me." I looked at him and he gave me a wink.

"Whatever Joshua."

"No, it isn't whatever; it's the truth." I left it at that and decided to let him get the last word.

I was a pro at cooking breakfast, so the food was done in less than 15 minutes. I served Joshua his plate and sat down to eat mine.

"Oh, I almost forgot to ask you, how did your doctor's appointment go?"

Looking at him, surprised, I answered, "It went okay."

I thought he had forgotten about it. I mentioned something to him about it and left it at that; I didn't think he would have remembered. One thing that we both agreed to keep in our relationship was honestly, straightforwardness, and commitment. If either one of us broke the promise, the relationship would be terminated.

"That's it? It was just ok?"

I really didn't like talking to Joshua about my mental situation. It made me so insecure and he worried a lot about it. I tell him all the time about how I think he will leave me for someone else because of it, but he tells me that he doesn't want any other. Suddenly, I lost my appetite; I put my fork down then thought about what I was going to say. There was silence for about half a minute before he concluded to break it.

"Is there a problem that I should know about? You know I want to know everything that is going on with you. I am not here to judge you or make you feel small. I'm here to support you and make you feel complete. I love you and I don't want anyone else. So tell me the truth, what's going on?" It sounded like the same old words he usually said before we discuss me, but I didn't mind them at all. I wanted to know he still cared.

"Well, the doctor changed my diagnosis."

"She did what?" Joshua asked, vexed.

"Yeah, she changed it."

"What is it?"

"Dr. Givins changed it to being Schizoaffective Disorder Bipolar Type."

"Is that like being schizophrenic and bipolar at the same time?" I looked at him with awe, for he knew without me telling him.

"Umm yeah, it is…how did you know?"

"I did some researching of my own when I was in jail."

"Oh, I'm impressed."

"Don't be. I really didn't read on anything called Schizo…whatever you called it. I just took it for what it sounded like. There are so many people that have your condition Samone, it's not even funny. You are not the only one who suffers from this. There are people that are worse off than you are; you should feel blessed."

"I understand what you are saying Joshua, but I don't feel blessed. If anything, I feel cursed right now."

"Why, because you can't change what happened to you? Everyone just about has something wrong with them; I have asthma. You don't see me complaining and trust me, there are people out there that do not know what asthma do to you and they fear it."

Love's Mirage

Ever since I've known Joshua, he has always been an optimistic person, either in a good or bad situation. The only thing that really got to him is being in jail; he hated his freedom being taken.

"I never told anyone this Samone, but one time I had an asthma attack and almost died."

I looked at him with shock, "What? Why did you wait so long to tell me something like that? What happened?"

"It's something that I try to forget but can't. It happened to me when I was about 14-years-old. I was outside playing football with my boys and suddenly, I couldn't catch my breath. The more I tried to breathe, the heavier my chest felt. I remember falling to the ground and being surrounded by my friends. I still can see their worried expressions so vividly within my mind till this very day."

I could tell that it still bothered him, for he looked at me with horrendous eyes and said, "Tyrone was there. He can tell you what happened; he was the one trying to coach me into breathing. I remember him telling me, *"Joshua, just clam down…try to take small breaths of air instead of large ones. You can do it."* I tried to do as he suggested, but no air was able to get to my lungs. So, I just laid there waiting for something like a miracle to happen. I guess someone in the neighborhood seen what happened and called an ambulance; I don't know because I had blacked out and was unconscious. When I awoke I was in the hospital greeted by my father, mother, and Tyrone. They had the room decorated with balloons and flowers stating to get well. That asthma attack was so bad that I had to stay in the hospital for one and a half weeks. You are the only person that I have ever told that story to and I made Tyrone swear never to tell anyone. Fortunately, for me he hasn't, that's why I love him like my very own brother," he smiled a boyish grin then preceded, "Samone, take that as a sign of me trusting you in sharing my past with you. I know I share everything about my life with you now but my past…well, I seem to have a problem with telling you about it."

"Why?"

"Because somehow it makes me feel insecure and I think you would leave me for someone else."

I looked at him with a smirk; I didn't know if I should have taken that remark seriously are sarcastic. I always said that to him and now he was using my very own words against me, how typical of him.

So, I asked him, "Did you mean that sarcastically? I mean, those words are often used by me."

He shrugged his shoulders and answered, "Take it in whichever way you wish, but know they are real."

"So, basically, you want me to take it seriously. That's all you had to say Joshua."

"Hopefully, my story made you feel somewhat better. I mean, I'm still here and living, thank God."

"Yes it did, thank you, because it made me feel a ton better." I stood up, leaned over the table, then kissed him.

"You are most welcome." I thanked him for opening up to me while clearing the table.

"…I really appreciated it. I know sometimes it can be hard to tell loved ones what's really on your heart for fear of what they may think, but let's both try not to let that stop us from being honest to one another, okay?"

"Okay," he said. He got up from the table and began to help me.

"Have you heard about Tyrone and Michelle?"

"Oh yeah, I knew about it before you or Michelle. Tyrone opened up to me about Michelle; he told me how much he "thinks" he loves her. I think he is rushing into it, but that's just my opinion."

"I know, I tried to tell the same thing to Michelle, but she got upset with me. She asked me to be her maid of honor."

"Did you agree?"

"Yeah, I told her I would love to be her maid of honor. I don't think she believed the "love" part in that sentence, though. When I told her I would do it, she gave me a sarcastic response of *"mmhhh sure you would."* I left it at that; I didn't want to take the chance to get in a more heated argument."

"Well, I hope Michelle is ready for Tyrone because he swears he loves her and honestly, I haven't heard or seen him get so excited with just talking about a woman. Every time her name is mention, he gets this glow in his eyes, it's beginning to become kind of spooky."

"Oh, so being in love is spooky to you?"

"No, I didn't mean it like that. I just meant to say that he is crazy in love with her. That's all. Samone, do you ever fear of getting hurt by me?" I looked at him while washing the dishes.

"Yes and no."

"What do you mean by yes and no?"

"Yes, because you scare me with your job occupation, no because you are so sweet and gentle to me that it makes me feel secure. I want you to know that your job scares me because you could end up getting hurt or go to jail for the rest of your natural life," I wiped my hands of dishes and turned Joshua's face to face my own, "you going to jail for life is horrifying to me. I would have no more you. I would have to start all over for love again. Joshua, I need you to promise me that you will stop. Not tomorrow but today, can you handle that?" He looked at me with intensive eyes.

"Samone, we have had this conversation before and what did I tell you? I told you that I am going to quit."

"I know you relayed the message to me, but you didn't tell me when. That is what I need to know now. When Joshua…when are you going to stop?"

"I'm being honest when I say this Samone…"

He took my face in his hands and whispered, "Soon as I make you my wife…that's when I will quit."

I had mixed emotions when he whispered that. At first, I thought it was a good answer because he was thinking of marriage with me. On the other hand, I didn't know when he planned to ask me to marry him; it could be years before he pops the question.

"Marriage?" I exclaimed, "do you really think we are ready for marriage any time soon? I'm looking for you to quit selling now and you are talking about marriage and then stopping. What is it about quitting that is so hard? I mean, all you have to do is get out of the game. Joshua, please throw your cards in." I could see the aggravation building within his facial expressions.

"Look Woman, I told you all I can about that. I can't quit right now and that's just that. If you can't see yourself with me as your husband, then maybe we should just call it quits now. I mean, I love you and I'm telling you that I want to marry you and all you are thinking about is me selling. I know what I do isn't right. I know I need to stop and I am, just give me time.

Damn, you are really starting to get on my nerves. Stop nagging me Samone!" He put the last dish in the dish rack and waited for me to reply.

When I didn't, he then replied, "Aren't you going to say something? You always have something to say."

I stood there, not knowing what to say. I didn't know if I wanted to respond rudely just as he did me. If I did, I knew it would be an argument. So, I didn't say anything. There was silence for about 3 minutes before he broke it by pleading with me to say something.

"I don't feel like talking to you right now. I've said all that I have to say for now."

When he saw that I was upset and gave him the silent treatment, it made the situation worst. He hated the silent treatment and he felt that we should speak our minds no matter what the situation was.

"Fine, if you don't want to talk to me, I'm leaving."

He stormed out of the kitchen and entered the bedroom. Like a lost puppy, I followed. I still had nothing to say to him, but I just wanted to watch him dress and make sure that he saw me angry before leaving. I also wanted him to take me to get my prescription, but since he was so upset, I didn't know. So I pushed my anger aside and decided to ask anyway.

"Joshua, will you take me to get my prescription?" It was the quickest I had ever seen him put his clothing on. He stopped tying his shoe to look at me. He looked at me with an annoyed expression.

"What? You want me to do something for you after you made me angry. I don't think so. Find your own ride."

I liked the way he was when he was upset at me. Don't ask me why, but I thought it was cute. He started mumbling things and I could tell he wasn't all that upset that he pretended to be. He was putting on a show because he wanted to get his way. He wanted me to be understanding about the whole drug situation and I wasn't having it.

"You know what? You better be glad I love you. Get dressed I will take you." He had his back to me, looking for his keys. I smiled to myself because I knew he was going to take me. I walked up to him and hugged him from the back.

"No, you better be glad I love you. I just hope you realize that." He turned around to face me.

"Samone, what if I told you when I expected to quit. Will you make a big deal about the timing?"

"I don't know. It depends on how long it will be, I guess."

"Well, in that case, I will leave you in suspense."

"Don't do that, tell me," I pleaded.

He smiled that gorgeous smile and replied, "I can't stay mad at you for too long. I'm glad you are my woman and all, but I'm not telling you when I thought of quitting. The next thing I know, you will be hounding me for an answer if I happen to break my word and we can't have that. I can just hear you now."

He began to focus on his thoughts and described my exact words to him, but he did it in a silly high pitched voice that totally did not sound like me. I couldn't help but laugh at his silliness.

"Oh Joshua, when are you going to quit? You told me you were going to quit this day and you still haven't. I must be a fool to be in love with you." He put on his watch and ended his expression of me with a…"blah blah, you know how you are Samone."

I just looked at him, for the words he spoke for me sounded something like me. I didn't want to admit it, but Joshua pretty much knew me. He always tells me that he has my mind and therefore, he has me. The hard part is accepting his words to be factual. After we finished discussing our argument and making up, he persuaded me to finish getting dressed. So, I put on my jeans and a cute neon green and yellow shirt that read, some girls have all the boys. I put my K Swiss's on and was finished dressing. I grabbed my keys, purse, and then we were out the door.

Once we were in the car, Joshua put on some Waymond Tisdale; he loved Jazz just like I did. I let out a laugh while thinking about how a thug was hip to Jazz.

Joshua didn't know what I was laughing at, so with a smile, he asked, "Why are you laughing?"

I smiled and said, "Do you really want to know?"

"Now that you have asked, yes. You make me want to know even more. So, tell me what it is?"

"Well, I was just thinking about how you like Jazz."

"Yeah, and why is that so funny?"

"Well, let's face it, Joshua you are a thug. Thug dudes usually don't listen to Jazz."

"And that is so funny to you, huh?"

"Yep."

"Cute Samone, I know a couple of thug dudes who love Jazz, I'm not the only one."

"I bet you do." He let out a laugh.

"You just won't leave me with the last word, will you?" I shook my head, no.

"You are something else, Ms. Grey, something else indeed."

We were on Riverside when we stopped at a red light and guess who pulled up beside us. It was Charles in his silver Impala. He looked over to see us and he gave a head movement up as to say what's up. I guess he didn't see me in the car at first, but I could see the irritation in his eyes as soon as he did. The light turned green and he spun off really fast while making smoke appear in the air. Joshua took off after him in a more decent manner.

"I wonder what his problem is," Joshua said.

"I don't know."

Deep inside, I knew what the problem was. Charles wanted me and he didn't know how to take me away from Joshua. He knew the type of man Joshua was and he feared to pursue any involvement in trying to obtain my love.

"As a matter of fact, I think Charles owe me some money," Joshua said out loud.

"Oh, really, how much do you think he owes you?" Joshua was still thinking out loud, for he did not hear anything I asked him.

"Yeah, he owes me…I got to get that money." I shook him on the shoulder.

"Joshua. Do you hear me talking to you?"

"Oh, uh…huh? I mean, what did you say?" He looked at me, then back at the road.

"I asked you how much money do he owe you?"

"Samone, I want you to know something."

I answered, "What's that?"

"You are really nosey." I punched him on the arm and he let out a laugh.

"I get it from you."

"No, you don't either."

As we entered Walgreens' parking lot, I noticed that there weren't many people, which was a good thing. I really didn't feel like waiting in line for 30 minutes to an hour. My cell phone rang as I was getting out of the car.

I answered the phone, "Hello. Hey Girl, what's up?"

"Hey Samone." I turned around to look at Joshua to see what he wanted.

"Could you hurry up this process? I have to be somewhere in an hour."

I had the phone on my ear and Michelle was talking to me at the same time Joshua was, so I just shook my head yes. The store was bare of people and Walgreens was the type of store that always had customers in it.

"No, I'm not busy…I'm just getting my medicine."

"I told you, Michelle that I was going to be off work today and tomorrow. Yeah, my boss was very understanding. I actually couldn't believe that she gave me these days off so effortlessly. Yeah, you can come through. I should be back home within 20 minutes."

"Ok. See ya' soon. Bye."

Walking as swiftly as possible, I made my way to the pickup line in the pharmacy area. I only had to wait for 15 minutes for the whole process to be over. With my medicine in hand, I looked around to make sure there was no one there that I knew. I exited the store and nearly skipped to the car. Michelle wanted to meet me at my house to discuss her wedding and to talk to me. I knew she wanted to express her feelings about the other night. I was ready for her.

"So, who was that on the phone?"

"Oh that was Michelle," I said as I was getting back into the car, "she wants to come over and hang out with me."

"Oh, well let's get you back home. I got 45 minutes to get where I need to go." I was about to ask him where he had to go, but I figured he had to go and visit his probation officer.

We zoomed down Riverside and he had me back at my apartment complex within 10 minutes.

"Ok, Baby I'll see you later." Joshua leaned over and kissed me.

I got out of the car and he was gone. It made me sad to see him leave for the day. I probably won't see him until later on that night. As I was headed toward my apartment, I noticed a body standing where my door was. It was Charles. I almost panicked because I thought about the possibility of Joshua finding him there.

"Charles, what the hell are you doing here?"

He had fire in his eyes, but he politely said, "I needed to see you. I saw you with Joshua and it made me mad as hell. I can't believe that you are still with him after the conversation we had."

"Umm, hold up Charles. I never told you that I was going to break up with Joshua and I also told you that I would give you a call." I brushed passed him to get to my door.

"I think you should really leave now Charles. It's not appropriate for you to be here."

"Not appropriate…Woman bring you ass here." He grabbed me by the arm and my prescription fell out of my hand. He stooped over and picked it up.

"What the hell is this?" He looked at me with concern and waited for an answer.

I stood there frozen not knowing what to say. Just when I was about to say something Michelle showed up. She had a surprised expression on her face. Charles didn't like Michelle because Michelle didn't like him. He really didn't have no beef with her but she made it obvious every time she seen him that she didn't care for him.

"What's up Samone." She didn't even speak to Charles; she ignored his presence.

"Hello to you too, Michelle."

"Oh, hello Charles. I thought I said hello to you.. my bad."

I noticed the brewing temperature rising within me and I thought I was about to have another panic attack. So I began to breathe in deeply and slowly. They both faced me and asked me was I okay. I nodded yes and told them I just needed something to drink.

"Well, I guess we will see you later Charles," Michelle said.

"Umm I didn't hear Samone tell me to leave Michelle, so just mind your own damn business."

"See, that's why I don't like your ghetto ass. You always getting smart with someone."

"Hold up. You are the one trying to dismiss me like I came over to see you or something."

He looked back at me and retorted, "You need to check your friend." I didn't want to get in between the argument so I just stood.

"No, Samone you need to check his ass before I do."

Charles gave me back my prescription and said, "Look, I'll call you later, I still want to know what's up." I took the medicine and opened my apartment door.

He turned in the direction of his car and left. When we got inside I told Michelle about herself.

"Now, you know you were wrong. Why you do that to him every time? Why do you get him so angry?"

"I did what I did because I wanted him to leave. And guess what, he left. I don't know why you are taking up for him. You don't belong with him; you belong with Joshua and that's that."

I just looked at her and shook my head. I had no words for her. There was no changing her mind; she was very stubborn at times.

"Michelle, he is still my friend. Just because he doesn't make the kind of money Joshua does, doesn't mean he is not right for me."

"So, what are you saying? You want to be with him?" Michelle looked at me with disbelief, "what was he doing here anyway? Did you invite him over here?"

"No, I didn't. He was already here when I got here, which I told him he shouldn't have done." I sat down across from where she was sitting.

"Do you feel better since you got that drink?"

"Yeah, Girl, I was about to have one of my panic attacks." She looked at me with concern.

"I sure hate that you go through those things. You are so strong to go through things like that and not complain about it. I admire you for that."

"Girl, don't do too much admiring because I have my days when I do complain. I just don't complain to everybody."

She quickly changed the subject, "But back to what we were talking about. That's kind of spooky for Charles to be popping up over at your place and you don't even be here."

"I know. He does it to try and break Joshua and me up. I'm worried because one day he is really going to catch Joshua over here and things are going to go down. You know Joshua has a temper."

"I know, Samone that's why I ran him off. What if Joshua thought y'all was really together doing something behind his back? Do you know how much trouble it would be for the both of you?"

I just sat there and inhaled all the propositions she was giving me. I then began to tune her out because it was just too much to think about.

"What if you and Joshua broke up?" That was the last thing I heard before I interrupted her.

"So, what did you want to talk about?" She stopped and gave me a dirty look.

"Samone, you know, you can be one rude woman at times. I was in the middle of a sentence."

"I'm sorry, but my head is beginning to hurt from talking about all the what-ifs. Can we just talk about something else?"

"Samone, that's all you had to say, instead of just rudely interrupting me. Well, I wanted to talk to you about the last time I was over here. You kind of dampened my spirit about marrying Ty, but you made me think. We have only been dating for six months now, which is such a short time to consider marriage. I told Ty what you said and he got upset. He told me that I shouldn't listen to you and that we can do whatever the hell we wanted to do."

"Why did he say that for? I never told you not to marry him; I just told you to think about it."

"Well, whatever you said made an impression on me. It made me think that I wasn't ready and that's exactly what I told Ty. Now, he is angry with both you and me."

"Why is he so angry? I mean, you are only considering to just wait a little longer."

"I know, but he feels that we are really ready now."

"I already knew that you wanted to talk about that before you even opened your mouth. I just thought you were going to tell me that you were angry about it. What made you change your mind about the whole situation?"

"About what?" she asked.

"About waiting."

"Oh, I just want to make sure he is the right man for me. There is no doubt in my mind that he is not cheating on me; I just want to make sure he is compatible with me."

"There you go, that's what I wanted to hear."

I smiled, listening to my friend tell me the good news. She was talking like she had sense. I'm really surprised that Michelle took my advice. I mean, the girl put on a show the last time she was over here.

"What do you mean, there I go?" I got up and hugged her.

"Well, Girl, you are talking with some sense; that's what. You have to understand, I only want the best for you and I want you to make sure that whoever he is that you decide to marry is the right one."

"So, tell me, Samone, how do you know if he is the right one? I mean, you are telling me all this and here you are dating the top dog of selling." I couldn't say anything, for she was right; I was dating the head negro in charge.

"Well, I don't have an answer to your question. All I know is that six months is such a short time to know someone thoroughly and you guys are talking about marriage. Marriage is another level, a level that I think you are just not ready for. I hope I don't offend you; I'm just trying to be honest with you. As far as for me, dating the as you would say, the "top dog," well, I don't know what to do with him."

"I know what you should do with him…marry him. Maybe then he will quit doing what he is doing. Y'all have been dating for two years now and according to you, that is plenty of time to know someone."

"To be honest, I don't know what to do with Joshua. Joshua is the biggest drug lord in Texas right now and I don't know if I should love him or hate him."

"I know what you mean Samone. I sometimes think about Ty selling drugs and it gets to me. I wonder why he just can't find a regular 9 to 5 kind of job. You know what it is right; they both want that fast money."

"You are definitely right about that. Until you said that, Michelle I thought you were okay with Tyrone selling; I didn't know you felt like that."

She looked at me like I were crazy and said, "Hell yeah, that shit bothers me. I can't believe you would think differently."

"I only thought that because you were itching to marry him in such a short time…that's all."

I could tell that I offended her; she started cursing. She usually starts to curse when she is either highly upset or is becoming upset.

"Yeah Girl, his selling does get to me…" Her tone level was once again normal.

"I once asked him to quit, but he got upset with me. He told me that he is going to ride till he die. What am I going to do Samone? At least Joshua is considering quitting for you, but Tyrone says he will never quit."

I didn't know what to tell her, so I told her the best thing that I could come up with, "Well, Samone you either are going to love him for better or worse, or you are going to have to leave him. If he is telling you that he will not change, I would take that into consideration. Don't ever think that you can change a man. I made that mistake a long time ago. If they change, it is probably on their own."

"You are telling me that a little too late. I already thought love would make him change. I have realized that my love is not enough to make him change." Her voice began to break as if she were about to cry, "Samone…" She grabbed my hand, "I think I may be pregnant. That is the other reason I wanted to talk to you."

"Uh-oh. Did you take a pregnancy test?"

"No, but I brought one, though. Do you know anything about pregnancy tests, because I didn't know which one to get, so I just grabbed this one." She took her purse and opened it to find the pregnancy test. I took the pregnancy test to examine it.

"Well, it says that you will get an accurate result, so I think it's fine."

Before she stood up to go to the bathroom, she began to cry. I got up from my seat and hugged her.

"Are you okay?"

"No, Samone I'm not okay. If I am pregnant…" She stopped speaking.

"I know it's hard for you to concentrate right now and really don't know what to do, but you are going to get through this. Who knows, this may very well change the outlook of life for the father to be. So take a deep breath, go down that hall and take that test." She wiped at her eyes, took in a deep breath, and did as I instructed her to do.

CHAPTER THREE

After about 20 minutes of waiting, she came out smiling.

"I take it that you are not?"

"Yep. I'm not pregnant!" She ran down the hall with such happiness and glee as she hugged me.

"I am so ecstatic that the results came back negative. I was so nervous the whole time I was in there waiting. Girl, you just don't know, when I saw one line on the applicator, my heart just lifted. Maybe one day, I will be ready for kids, but for right now, I know that I am not."

I looked at her while she broke out with the Cabbage Patch dance. I let out a laugh.

I thought to myself, *"Oooh, my friend is so silly at times."*

The next thing I knew, she had me doing the cabbage patch with her. After all the dancing, laughing, and singing we sat down out of breath.

"You know what Samone?"

"What?"

"You are so silly. Why did your face have to be all scrunched up while you were dancing?"

I let out another laugh and said, "Oh, you know that's the way I do it. That face helps me get my best moves displayed.

"Mmmpph, like I said, you are so silly. I'm glad though because you make me laugh."

"Am I here to entertain you? Do you expect me to be your clown?"

"Umm, I know. I know what movie you got that off of."

"Michelle, you better, it happens to be off of one of your so call favorite movies." She let out a giggle and proceeded with the answer.

"You got that off of Goodfellas."

"Yep. Good job."

After I said the phrase, I realized I got the wording wrong, but I didn't bother trying to fix it because she knew what I was talking about. She clicked on the television and began to surf the channels. I left her there while I went to put my prescription away, which I then began to remember the facial expression Charles had when he saw it. It was kind of scary.

Then, his words began to replay in my mind, *"What the hell is this?"*

I know he will definitely bring it up again the next time he either sees me or talks to me. I must be ready with an answer, but I still don't know what to say. Maybe I should just tell him the truth. Naw, then he would think of me as some kind of crazy person and that I can't have. To tell you the truth, when I saw him standing at my doorstep, my heart skipped a beat. It felt good in a weird sort of way. He cared about me so much that he decided to surprise me with his presence.

"Samone!" Michelle yelled.

"What are you doing back there? It doesn't take that long to put your medicine up."

I snapped out of my thoughts and mustered up a response, "Girl, I'm coming. What do you need me for anyway?" Closing the medicine cabinet, I looked in the mirror and smile.

I told myself, *"You go girl."*

"What are you doing in here?" Michelle was now in the bathroom with me looking concerned as before.

"Nothing. I was just about to come back into the living room. Man, can't a Sista' just get some privacy around here without being questioned?"

She shook her head no, "Not as long as I'm around, besides, I was just making sure you were alright. You do remember that you were about to have another panic attack, right?"

I exhaled with attitude, "Yes, I remember all of that, but as you can see, I am alright. Now, please stop worrying so much. If anything, you could be making me something to eat." She looked at me with a raised brow.

"Do you really expect me to cook? Come on now, don't try to be funny with me. You know that I can't cook all that good right now. It is in the near future that I will begin to experiment with some food, pots, and pans. Now, with that being said, what are we going to have for lunch?"

"Umm, I don't feel like cooking, so I guess we are going to have to starve."

She began to plead with me, "Ahh, come on Samone. Make us something to eat."

"Michelle, you are 19-years-old. I think it is way past the time in which you should know something about cooking. You should be ashamed of yourself and besides, I know you know how to cook something. You are just pretended, so I will do all the slaving around here. I cooked last time and you are definitely no new company, so I suggest you do the cooking this time."

She gave me a pouting look and said, "Please."

I shook my head no, "Nope, not a chance."

She picked up my telephone and began to dial numbers, "I guess we will have to eat some pizza because I'm not going to cook neither. Umm, yes, I can hold."

I picked up the remote and turned it to one of my favorite noonday shows, "The Jerry Springer Show."

"Samone, what kind of toppings you want your pizza?"

"Get me my favorite."

"Ok," I overheard her say the order, "…yeah, a medium supreme pizza with extra cheese. Yes, that's all. Thanks."

"Mone, I don't know why you like to watch that show. You know it's all pretend."

"It may be, but it's entertaining me like it's supposed to."

She smacked her lips and said under her breath, "The things people will watch and do for entertainment." I was going to respond to her smart remark, but I decided not to.

"I am truly starved. How long did they say the pizza would take?"

"They told me that it would be here within 45 minutes to an hour."

I started complaining and Michelle just ignored me because I always complained about how hungry I was when I was hungry. I complained and complained and then complained more.

"Samone, would you shut it up. You are really getting on my nerves right now. They will get here when they get here." By this time, she knew I was messing with her, for I heard it in the tone of her voice.

"But Michelle, I'm so hungry. I need something to eat right now."

"Go into the kitchen and find something then, with your silly self. I know you are just getting on my nerves for no apparent reason. Oooh, you are a piece of work."

I got up from my couch, went to where she was sitting, and began to lean on her as if I were dying of hunger.

"Help me Michelle. Help a Sista out." She began to laugh.

"Gone Samone."

She pushed me trying to get me off, but she did not succeed and I had an advantage over her. So, I was not going anywhere.

"Michelle help me..." I began to drool at the mouth. She looked at the saliva that was about to fall on her.

"Yuck...Samone, stop playing and get off of me. You are truly sick."

"I know...that's why I take medicine."

I got up from leaning on her and sat up straight. I got quiet, then put on a serious expression.

"Samone, now you know I didn't mean it like that."

"Uh-huh, sure you didn't. You really hurt my feelings." I put my head in my lap to hide my face so that she could not see the fake tears.

"Samone stop playing around." I then began to make fake sobbing noises.

"Fine, I hope I did hurt your feelings. Because you are hurting mine right now with all this faking." I kept crying.

"Ugh, stop it. I was only joking."

I picked my head up and smiled, "I know."

She gave me a punched on the arm and said, "You know what? You should really consider going into acting classes because you really be putting on a show."

"Do you really think I could make it?" I asked sarcastically.

Just as she was about to answer me, the doorbell rang. I jumped up and down and faked a scream, then whispered, the pizza is here.

"Sit down Samone, really sit your ass down. You are getting carried away here." I sat down as she commanded.

Michelle opened the door and to our surprise, it wasn't the pizza man, it was Tyrone.

"Tyrone," Michelle said with a high pitched voice, "what are you doing here?"

"Can I come in," he said. She moved out of his way and he entered the door.

"I came by to talk to Samone about you and me." He turned his attention to me. He looked as if he just got fired from his job.

"Why do you wish to speak to me," I asked.

I stood up from the couch to beckon for him to sit.

He rejected my offer to a seat with the words of, "Nah, I won't be here long." After he rejected my offer, I knew that this was going to be a bad conversation.

"Just what I needed," I thought to myself.

"Why is it every time I find a woman I love her friend get in between our business?" He started to shake his head and then rubbed it with his left hand.

Michelle meanwhile was sitting down with this disbelief expression. I guess she could not believe that he was actually over here confronting me about their relationship.

"I don't understand it. I mean, I do all I can to make my woman happy and she always ends up listening to her friend."

"Tyrone, I don't know the conversation you and Michelle had, but I do know this…I only told her that she should wait a little longer. That's all."

"I know that's what you said…I remember those exact words of yours. Trust me; you do not have to repeat them. I know them by heart. I mean, they have actually been playing in my head all day."

Both of my eyebrows rose with concern. I knew this man was about to flip out. I just didn't know if he was planning on doing any harm. I also wondered if Michelle knew what was going to happen. I began to prepare myself for the worst. He walked up on me till he was in my face.

"You really need to stay out of grown folks business with your ugly ass." My mouth dropped.

I couldn't believe this man was actually this mad over a little advice. I didn't know what to say, so I just stood there.

"You can close your mouth before I put something in it." He motioned for me to look down and I saw a gun.

I thought to myself, *"What was that for?"*

Michelle was trying to back him up and she managed to get in between him and I.

"Baby, just calm down." I guess Michelle wasn't as dumb as she looked over there sitting down.

"What were you thinking about when you decided you were going to bring a gun into my house? Were you thinking of using it on me?"

The doorbell rang again, this time, it was the pizza man. All eyes went to the door.

"Who is that?" Tyrone asked Michelle. Michelle was still standing in between us.

"That's the pizza man," she whispered. My eyes then turned back to Tyrone.

"What are you planning to do with that gun Tyrone?"

"If you keep in Michelle and my business, you will see."

"Is that a threat?" The doorbell rang again.

"Baby, what's wrong with you? How could you even think about harming Samone? She is my…"

"I know who the hell she is…fuck her. I told you that I was going to do this. You must not have believed me, huh? I told you Michelle. I told you." I looked at Michelle, who had tears in her eyes.

"Nah Baby, I didn't believe you. Could we just talk about this some more?"

I was in disbelief at this moment in my life. My best friend knew that her man was planning on threatening me with a gun, and she didn't bother to let me know. I couldn't believe this. I sat down with little air in my lungs. By this time, the pizza man walked off. I guess he figured no one was at home, but I know he heard the commotion going on. Tyrone pushed Michelle to the side.

He then hovered over me and said, "If you ever open your mouth to speak negatively about me to anyone…I will kill you. That means Joshua and Michelle," he looked over at Michelle, who was now crying fountains of tears, "…and you better tell me if she do tell anybody. She's your best friend, right and y'all tell each other everything, right, well, now you have something to talk about among one another." He then turned his attention back to me. "I mean it, Samone if you tell Joshua about this…you and Michelle's life is in jeopardy." With that, he stormed out of the door.

Both of us were in total shock and we felt helpless. I thought about how just a few minutes ago, I was joking around and in the twinkling of an eye my life had been threatened. Joshua needed to know this information. I pulled out my cell phone and searched for his number.

Michelle looked up from her wet hands and said, "What are you doing? Didn't you hear what he just said?"

I pretended not to hear her and kept searching. I found his number and dialed it. It rang five times before it went to his voice mail. Michelle, meanwhile, got up and snatched the cell phone out of my hand.

"You are going to listen to me Samone. My life is in his and your hands. If you tell anybody, we are dead!"

I looked at her with a disgusted, angry, and a hurt look. She killed my heart. My best friend held out on me when it counted. All of my emotions of what just happened started to react within me at the same time. I was happy because I was still alive, I was sad because my life had been threatened, I was hurt because my friend betrayed me, and I was mad because my prescription wasn't equipped to handle all of this commotion at once. I tried to keep my composure and wait it through, but I then began to have rushing thoughts and my emotions being out of control.

I started crying and said through tears, "I'm hurting Michelle...help me."

"Wake up Baby. Wake up." I woke up to the voice of my beloved boyfriend. I don't know how long I was out, but I saw Joshua's concerned face looking down at me when I opened my eyes.

"What is going on? How long have I been out?" I looked at Michelle, who had this scared horrific look on her face that it made me think that I did some weird things.

"...did I do anything weird? What happened?"

"Just calm down, Samone. We will answer all your questions as soon as you relax," Joshua expressed with a soothing voice. He began to stroke my face with the back of his hand.

"When did you get here?"

"I got here about two hours ago. Michelle called me up, saying that you had another panic attack and that she didn't know what to do. I came as soon as I finished my deal, which I was just about finished when she called. I hate seeing you like this. Did you take your medicine?" I looked at him with no expression and he waited for the answer.

"Samone, are you okay? Did you just hear what I asked you?"

"Yes, I heard you, I know what you said. No, I haven't taken my medicine yet because it's not time yet." I tried to sit up, but Joshua had his arm around my waist so that I couldn't get up.

"No, Sweetie, don't try to get up. You need your rest."

"I'm cool Baby, trust me. Let me up." He moved his arm so that I could sit up.

Michelle came closer to the bed, for she was just standing in the doorway, looking as if she was lost. To tell you the truth, I didn't want to have anything else to do with her after what had happened today.

"Are you okay Samone?" Michelle asked.

I gave her a dry smile and said, "Yes, I'm fine."

"Well, you really scared me a while ago. I didn't know what to do." At that time, I wasn't thinking about what I did, but now she had my curiosity about what happened.

"What happened?"

"Umm, you don't need to remember the things you did...they will only make you feel like you are crazy." I looked at Joshua and wondered why she had just made that comment.

"Will someone just tell me the damn truth of what happened?" I was starting to get irritated by their behavior.

"Baby, I really don't think you want to know what you did."

"How do you know what I would like to know? Are you in my head?" He got up from the bed and went over to where Michelle was.

"Ok, Michelle tell Samone what happened. Don't leave anything out."

"Before I start, Samone do you remember anything?" I didn't really want to hear anything she had to say, for she might lie.

"Well…" I sat on the edge of the bed.

"…I remember some things, but everything is not clear." Michelle looked at Joshua, who had encouraging eyes for her to go on and tell what happened.

"Go ahead Michelle, tell her what you told me."

"Wait a minute," I said.

"What?" they both replied. I rubbed my head and announced that my head hurt.

Joshua walked over to me and wrapped his arms around me and said, "My poor Baby. After all that you have been through today. You really do need to rest and we can talk about this at a later time."

"Nah, I want to know now what is going on. By the way, what time is it?"

"It is 7 o'clock," Michelle said.

"7? It feels like it is later than seven."

"That's because you have been sleeping for a long while. Joshua is right; maybe we need to talk about this a little later when you are feeling better."

I stood up while shaking my finger and head no, "No, Michelle I would like to know what you told Joshua." I gave her a stern look that made her shy like a child.

I looked to my right and Joshua's expression was confusion. He looked as if he wanted to yell out what in the hell is going on.

"Why are you so afraid of speaking Michelle?" Joshua asked.

"I know. Why is it so hard to just tell me what you said?" Michelle began to cry.

Both Joshua and I were confused as to why she was crying. I mean, I had an idea as to why she was crying, but Joshua didn't. Michelle and I both had a good reason to cry. Our lives could have been taken in a heartbeat, but yet, we were still living only to keep it a secret. I don't know how long I can keep something like that bottled up inside me.

"Will you both stop pressuring me to speak? Maybe I don't want to speak right now. Maybe, I just need some time to myself."

I could tell Joshua was becoming irritated by the way his closed mouth was twitching. Joshua lifted both hands out of frustration at Michelle and agreed to tell what happened.

"Fine, I'll tell you what she said. She told me that you had a hallucination that Tyrone wanted to kill you. She said that you were so sure that he was in this apartment today and that you saw him. She also told me that you imagined him having a gun and that he threatened you with it. That's what she told me."

My mouth gaped. I was so flabbergasted with what he told me that it left him concerned.

"You must tell me Samone if this is not at all true."

I looked at Michelle, who was pleading with her eyes for me to go along with her story.

"Samone, you don't remember the things you were doing, do you?" Michelle asked. I sat down with my hand on my chest.

"Don't remember. Don't remember," I replied.

"Well, Baby, do you remember anything?" Joshua sat next to me on the bed.

Some way or fashion I had to pretend that I wasn't upset. The truth of the matter is that I am very angry. I couldn't believe that Michelle would just lie about me having a hallucination and especially to something to that extreme degree. I mean, she actually made it seem like I would be lying if I told the truth. I thought about putting myself in her shoes for a few minutes but then realized that I didn't want to be anything like her, even if it was for just a few minutes. Damn her, why couldn't she just tell the truth. Why did she have to lie?

"Well, I remember somewhat of what Michelle said to be true. The rest of it, I don't remember." Michelle exhaled with relief.

"...but Michelle wasn't Ty over here for just a little while. I mean before I had a panic attack?" She looked at me with an attitude.

"Oh, now that you mentioned it, he was over here for just enough time to drop off some money to me." Joshua leaned in and gave me a kiss and hug.

"I'm glad that some of it is coming back. When you remember it all, just let me know all the details. By the way, I called your mother and told her what happened and she wants you to call her as soon as you get the chance. I swear your mother made it seem like it was my fault or something. She was pressuring me to tell her what happened. I couldn't because at that time

I didn't have all the details, so I was only able to tell her what I knew, and it definitely wasn't enough. She was going to swing by, but I assured her that everything was okay. I told her that Michelle was here helping me. Denise told me that she was going to tell Dedra to swing by, but she hasn't shown up yet."

I just listened to all that he had to say, but my mind started drifting off to other thoughts. The whole incident of the gun replayed in my mind again and again. Then I started thinking about Michelle and her big-time lies. She had great gumption to make up something like that. It just blew my mind that I actually went along with it. At least for now, that is. I do plan to tell Joshua or Charles what he did to me. Tyrone couldn't get away with this, not in the least. He was going to pay; he must pay for what he did to me. I don't know what Michelle is thinking about. She can't pretend for the rest of her life that it didn't happen. She had her way for now. I just need more time to come up with a plan. A plan that wouldn't put either one of our lives in danger.

I hugged Joshua and told him, "Thanks for calling my mother. I know Dedra hasn't shown up but has she called?" I cut Joshua off in the middle of his sentence, and he let me know that he was irritated by it.

"Samone...you know what...never mind." I guess he had sympathy for me because of what happened. Knowing him, it would have been a different story if things we better.

"Well, I'm going to the living room so you two can have your privacy."

"Thank you," I said in disgust.

She left the room at peace, so it seemed to me, but I wasn't at peace. I was very disturbed by emotions and thoughts. I sat there speechless as to what to say to Joshua while we had this time to speak.

"How are you feeling?" he asked.

"I'm fine," I lied.

"It seems to me that you and Michelle know more things than you are telling me. She came up with such an elaborate story. At first, I didn't believe her; I didn't want to believe her. *I mean, Ty is not that type of man. He wouldn't hurt something or someone I love, would he?*" He was thinking out loud more to himself than he was speaking to me.

I quickly intervene, "What do you think about Joshua? You know your friend better than anyone."

"I know I do, but lately he has been acting real strange when your name comes into the conversation." I was really surprised to hear that.

"Oh, really? Like how does he act?"

"I don't know how to explain it. It's…it's like he gets this look within his eyes that isn't pleasant and he quickly changes the subject. I mean, he does this every time." Now I was frightened for my life.

My own boyfriend has seen the anger Ty has against me. I couldn't believe the whole situation. I mean, all I did was give some advice to my "suppose" to be best friend. Who would have thought my words would have such a huge effect on someone.

"Joshua, should I be worried? I mean, you just told me that you friend has anger toward me."

He looked at me with worry in his face, "I don't know. He has done his dirt in the past, but he has never come up against me. This whole situation is making me look at him in a different light. I guess I will have to keep my eyes on him more. Try not to worry about him, though Samone."

"What about Michelle? How has he been acting when you mention her name?"

"Oh, he still gets delighted and overjoyed. He really loves her. Samone, what did you do to get him so upset with you?"

Not knowing if Joshua already figured things out, I lied to him, "I don't know." He looked at me as if he knew I was lying.

"Are you sure you don't know?"

I hated lying to him, but how could I tell him the truth just now, "Yes, I'm sure."

"Ok…Samone, I have given you a chance to tell the truth on anything you may be hiding. I just hope you are not lying to me about things. I got the strangest feeling that you are lying to me, though, but I can only go off of what you tell me. So, I'm going to leave it at that."

"I'm not lying to you Joshua…I told you what I know that happened."

"Yeah, you may have, but it seems to me that something is up and it hasn't come down yet." I leaned over to hug Joshua, but he pushed me away from him.

I struggled to understand what his reason was for doing that, "What is that about? You don't want to hug me now are something?" At first, Joshua didn't say anything; he just looked at me.

"I'm glad that you are doing better than what you were doing, God knows if something had happened to you, I would have been devastated, but I choose not to hug you because I know you. I know that you are hiding something from me. I can see it all in your eyes and over your face. You are really trying to pretend that you don't remember everything when you know you do. Just quit pretending and tell the truth."

I don't know how much longer I will be able to keep this man occupied with what I tell him. He is really digging deep and I know if anyone digs deep, they are bound to find something. Until I'm able to come up with a plan, I have to continue with the lie Michelle made up.

"Look Joshua; I'm telling you what I know…" The knock on the door interrupted my lie and I was relieved.

"Who is it?" I asked.

"It's me, Dedra can I come in?"

Joshua was bent over with his head in his hands. I wanted to make sure everything was cool enough between us before I told her to enter, but it looked to me that he didn't care.

"Yeah, come on in."

I got up from the bed and stood in one place until she came in. She entered the door with a huge smile on her face.

"Hey Girl, how are you doing?" She walked over to where I was and gave me a big bear hug.

"I'm doing okay."

"That's good. Now, I can call Mama and tell her that you are doing well. She is worried about you, you know?"

"Yeah, I know. I'm going to call her in a few minutes." Dedra turned her attention to Joshua, who was standing with a fake smile.

"Hey, what's up Joshua?"

"Aww, nothing much…just worrying about your sister." She walked over to him and gave him a friendly hug.

"I hope she is not worrying you too much. Nobody wants you to get stressed around here."

"Nah, it's nothing I can't handle."

"Hey, is Michelle still in there?" I asked.

"Yeah, she was watching T.V. before I came in here, but I don't know what she is doing now."

I left the two of them alone to go and find out if Michelle was still in the house. I found her lying on the couch, flipping the channels. It didn't seem like she was watching anything. It was more like the T.V. was watching her.

"Michelle, are you okay?" I asked. She sat up and shook her head, no.

"I'm sorry about lying," she whispered. She began to cry and her sobs were soft.

I didn't want to tell her that I was cool with what she did, because she made me look like a crazy person. I can only imagine the details that she told him. I know that I have a condition, but dang, she didn't have to encourage lies about the tragedy that happened today. This kind of drama will make anyone go insane. I don't know how I am handling all of this.

So instead of saying, it's ok, I said, "I'm sorry you had to lie. You made me look like a fool."

"No, I didn't…really. If you think about it, it makes perfect sense. Come on now Samone, don't be like that. Try to put yourself in my shoes for a moment. My life is resting in the hands of your words and Ty's decision."

"I know that Michelle," I walked over and sat down next to her, "I know what kind of trouble we are both in. That's why we need to tell someone. We can't just let Tyrone get away with this." She stood up.

"Just stop right there, that's how we got into this trouble in the first place. You always come up with some advice I just don't need at the time. I love you Samone, like you are my own flesh and blood sister, but you got to realize that this is a delicate situation and I'm going to handle it in that way. You got to put that fire of anger out. Let things resolve within themselves."

Amazed out of disbelief, I said, "I can't do that. I can't. I love you too, but you hurt me today. You knew all along what he was planning to do and you said nothing. You just pretended that everything was okay. How could you have done that?" Just then, my sister and Joshua came into the living room.

"What's going on in here?" Joshua asked.

"Yeah…why are y'all whispering?" Michelle and I both needed to finish this conversation but it would definitely have to be at different time. She looked at me; I looked at her, she opened her mouth to speak.

"Oh umm…we uh."

"We didn't notice that we were whispering. Besides that, we were just having a conversation about what happened today. I just am glad when all of this is over and we are back to normal."

"Whew…I know what you mean," Michelle said.

"I hate to be the one to bring the topic up again, but what happened? I'm still at a loss as to what happened."

"Well, maybe I should ask y'all what y'all were talking about because I left y'all in there for at least five minutes before y'all came out." They both shied with movement that showed them being uncomfortable.

"Well, we were talking about how mama got upset and began to blame Joshua for today's event."

Joshua cut in and said, "Yeah, and Dedra was filling me in on her studies in school. Can't you believe it Baby? Your sister is at the top of her class?"

I don't know what they were really talking about in there, but it really changed the thought process of Joshua, for he was actually smiling. Before I left the room, he was agitated.

"I know. She is always excelling in school; I am truly happy for my sister." My sister was smiling as I complimented her.

"Thanks, Sis." She walked over and hugged me.

"Congratulations Dedra, I didn't know you were so smart," Michelle said.

"Thank you, Michelle and everyone. I'm just glad that the Lord has blessed me with the mind that I got."

I guess she thought I would get offended by what she said because she glanced my way. I smiled to let her know that I was okay with what she said. I can't stand when people treat me different than what they used to. I mean, back in the day, she wouldn't have thought two seconds about what she said. It seems like since I've been diagnosed, that's how everyone has been treating me like and I hate it. It only reminds me that I am. I just wish things were back like they use to be before I became this way. I wouldn't have to be treated like a nutcase.

"So, has everyone eaten, because I am starved," Joshua announced.

"I ate before I came over here, so I'm fine."

"Are you sure Dedra, because I can order us a pizza?" Michelle asked.

I thought to myself, *"Is that all she knows how to do? Besides, the pizza place might not want to come back over here, after what happened today."*

"Yes, I'm sure. I just came over here to make sure Samone was alright."

"Don't tell me you are already planning to leave, are you?" I asked.

"Umm, well..."

"I was thinking about going out to dinner. You know, a sit-down type of thing," Joshua added.

"You can't leave yet...I want you to stay a little longer."

"Well, I guess I can," she said with hesitation.

"You know, I was thinking about Chili's, maybe we should go there and eat."

I ignored Joshua because I knew he was ignoring us. He was too busy thinking about his stomach than to hear what we were trying to say. I didn't blame him because we weren't discussing much. To tell you the truth, I was hungry myself.

"Ok, Joshua we get you; you are hungry, we know," Michelle said.

"Good. At least someone has heard my cry." He gave me eye contact as he said it.

"Ok, Baby let's go and feed you," I soothed. I reached over and gave him a kiss and hug.

"Are you sure you can stay because it sounded like you hesitated there for a minute?"

"Sure, I can stay. I just thought you didn't need me anymore."

"Girl sit down somewhere...now you know I need you. You are my blood."

She laughed, "You sit down somewhere. How about dem' apples?"

"Ah, so you are taking my very own phrases and are using them against me?"

"Yep."

"Michelle, are you coming with us?"

"You know what, I don't think I can make it, Joshua."

Love's Mirage

"Oh, and why not? Tyrone need you or something?"

"Umm yeah, he needs me." She quickly put on her shoes. She then grabbed her purse and pursued to the front entry.

Turning back to face us, she said, "Sorry I couldn't make it, but Tyrone called and he said he needed to talk to me about something." We caught our eyes.

"…I will call you later, okay."

"Ok. See you later." With that, she closed the door behind her.

"Aw man, I really wanted her to join us so I wouldn't be the third crowd."

"That's no way to look at the situation. You are invited to a wonderful evening with the two of us," Joshua explained.

"Yeah, you should feel lucky," I added.

"Whatever. Are we going to go or what?" my sister asked.

"Man…you must be hungry again or something. You are rushing us and things, just calm down," I said. She gave me an irritated facial remark.

"Oh my goodness…I almost forgot I got to call Mama."

"Oh, don't worry, you can call her while we are at the restaurant."

I asked my sister, "Dedra, do you think that would be wise? I mean, Joshua may not know what he is talking about."

"Yeah, Girl it's cool. Just get your stuff so that we can go." I walked to my bedroom and put my opened toed shoes on. Returning back to the living room, I found Dedra and Joshua laughing their heads off.

Grabbing my keys, I asked, "What is so funny?"

Still laughing, my sister said, "Oh, Joshua just told me about how one of his boys slipped and fell in Chili's one day."

"Oh yeah, you are going to have to fill me in on the story Joshua."

"I will. Let's go first, though; I'm starved."

While outside, my sister said, "I think we should both drive because I have to meet someone soon. I think it would be inconvenient if you would have to bring me way back over here."

Both Joshua and I faced one another and then replied, "Oh, so you are meeting up with your man?"

"Yep," she said with her head held high, "…and I'm proud of it."

"Okay…ok, that's fine." He assured.

We were stuck in traffic for about half an hour before we made it to another obstacle of Chili's parking lot. Cars were parked everywhere and cars were trying to find a parking place like we were. It took about 15 minutes before both cars could find a parking place.

Once out the car, my sister said to us, "I was about to give up. I'm glad someone finally left." I glanced at her while walking toward the entrance.

"I bet that's not the end of waiting for us." We all looked at the everlasting line before us.

"Are we sure we want to wait for a table?" she asked.

"I'm just that hungry to wait. I don't care how long the line is. I have wanted Chili's for a while now and that's what I'm gonna' get." We both looked at him with dissatisfaction.

Personally, I really didn't feel like waiting that long in line for Chili's. I was willing to have dinner elsewhere, but no, Joshua just had to have Chili's.

"I guess I'm willing to wait for at least half an hour."

"Me too."

"Samone, you are willing to leave me up here by myself? What kind of girlfriend are you?" He gave me a little shove so that I ended up off his arm. I grabbed his arm back to me.

"Uh-huh…get off of me." Dedra took all the action in and just smiled. She and I both knew that he was playing.

"Aw, don't be like that Joshua. You know that I love you."

"No, you don't. You want to leave me up here by myself to have dinner alone," he smiled.

"There is the smile I've been waiting to see all night. I just love your smile Joshua." Saying that to him made him smile even more.

"Stop Samone. You are making me blush and I'm hardcore. I'm not supposed to be smiling so hard." All three of us started smiling a huge smile.

We made into the entrance and noticed people sitting, eating, and talking galore. I just watched in amazement how the waiters and waitresses were doing their jobs hurriedly. It seemed as if they were wearing skates the way they were gliding by.

"Good evening. How many?" the hostess asked.

"Three."

"Would you like to sit in the smoking or non-smoking area?"

"Non-smoking." He handed Joshua an alert device to let us know when our table was ready.

"The wait will be at least 45 minutes." I looked at Dedra and she looked disappointed.

"Ok, thank you."

I turned around to look for us a place to sit while we waited. There were no seats available. I guess that was the reason for the waiting of people outside.

"Do y'all want to go outside and see if there are seats outside?" Both Joshua and Dedra looked at me like I had asked an awful question.

"Umm, I think not," she said.

"I have to agree with Dedra." I couldn't tell what the problem was with waiting outside. I mean, the weather was inoffensive.

"Well, what do y'all suggest? What, standing here in the middle of the way?" Dedra led us to an area that allowed three people to stand.

"This is a shame. I don't know if I want to wait here this long y'all. I mean, I have to be somewhere. I don't know if I will have time to eat."

"Well, we understand if you leave."

"Ok…I just wanted to tell y'all that before I left. I didn't want there to be any hard feelings."

"Oh no…we understand that you want to meet up with your man."

"I'm glad, Samone…I'm really glad you do."

"We both do. And who is this man anyway?"

"Umm, Samone don't you got to call Mama…" she cut me off.

"Oh yeah, I do have to call her, but I want to hear about this man you are now dating."

There was silence and with that silence, I started to think about the events that took place earlier that day. I started to think about the real reason why Michelle didn't dine with us. Doesn't she know that I could easily tell both Joshua and Dedra the truth of what happened? She left me the opportunity to do just that. Now the question is, shall I take it? If I did, I knew that there was a possibility that Michelle could die and I didn't want that hanging around my neck. To tell you the truth, I still have love for

Michelle. She was just put in a situation that got out of hand. I had to think like that to keep my saneness. I just couldn't bear the thought of her being involved with Tyrone planning to kill me. Then the question would be for what? Maybe it was for suggesting that they should take their time? No, that couldn't be the case. Honestly, I think there is another reason for him doing what he did to me and I'm going to find out. It just didn't make sense to me that he would do that. I have known Tyrone for at least two years now, and he wouldn't just flip out over something like that, but he did. I will never forget the image of Tyrone when he showed me that gun. I will never forget the fierceness in his eyes and his voice. He put on a good show and he made me wake up. People are not always who you think they are. Just when you think you know someone; they change on you. It's scary to think about, but here I was laughing and joking as if nothing happened. I wondered how I would be if my sister and man wasn't here for me right now. I wondered what Michelle was doing and what she must be thinking. She should have stayed with us. Maybe then she wouldn't be in danger of running into Tyrone.

CHAPTER FOUR

"Umm, hello. Earth to Samone. What are you thinking about?" I blinked my eyes to come back to the realization of my surroundings.

"Oh…umm, what? What did you say?"

"I asked you, are you going to call Mama now?"

"Yeah, I am. I'm sorry about that y'all. I was in deep thought."

"We know that. What were you thinking about?" Joshua asked.

"Oh, umm nothing. Just what happened earlier today." Joshua tried to soothe me with a hug.

"Try not to think about it. You were doing so good. It's okay. Things are going to be just fine." I pulled out my cell phone while he was still holding me.

"Thank you, Sweetie I needed to hear that." He pulled back to see what I was doing.

"Yeah, you better go ahead and call your mother. She will be saying I kept you from calling." I dialed my mother's number and she answered on the second ring.

"Where have you been? I have been so worried about you."

"Hello to you too Mama. I'm doing good. I'm here with Dedra and Joshua waiting in line at Chili's." Joshua left my side to go and talk with Dedra.

"Well, I'm glad you finally decided to call me. I talked with that ole boyfriend of yours earlier today. I should have gone over there, but I couldn't. I still had children that I was watching."

"I understand Mama." The lights went off on the alert device and it was time for us to sit down and eat.

"So how are you feeling now? Are you still having rushing thoughts?"

I was never deceptive to my mother, so I proceeded with the truth, "Yeah, a lil' bit, but nothing I can't handle."

"Did you take your medicine? When do you go back to the doctor? How long do you have off at your job?"

"Hold on Mama, with all the questions."

"Aw, Baby I'm just trying to find out what's going on with you; that's all." I followed the bodies to the table while I answered my mother's questions.

"Yes, I have been taking my old prescription, but I received a new prescription today, so I will now be taking that. I go back to the doctor two weeks from now and I have two days off until I'm expected back to work." I sat down and menus were given to us.

"Oh, okay…are you sure you are fine?"

"Yes, Mama I'm fine."

"Well, okay. Imma' let y'all eat and I will just chat with you later. I love you."

"Ok, Mama…and I love you too."

"Bye."

"Bye." I closed my flip phone and inserted it back into my purse.

"Well, that was a short conversation," my sister said.

"I know. Mama understood that we are in the process of eating dinner."

"Oh."

"Now see that didn't take too long, did it, Dedra?"

"Did what take too long?"

"Getting our table." Joshua looked up from the menu and smiled with satisfaction. The waitress came back to our table and asked if we were ready to order.

Our eyes met and I stated, "I would like a glass of water for starters."

"Me too," agreed my sister.

"Do you have sweet tea?"

"Yes, we do Sir. Would you like that?"

"Yes, I would. Thanks."

"You all take your time and I will be back with your drinks." She gave us a pleasant smile and left.

"I like her, she is nice. I think we should give her a good tip. What do y'all think?"

"I don't know just yet, Samone. Let's give her time to show us what she is made of."

"I don't know if I will be here with y'all to give her a tip."

"You may as well not order anything then. You speak as if you really need to be leaving right now."

"Honestly, I do. I have to make a stop at my apartment on the other side of town, take a shower, get dressed, and then head out to our special spot we hang out at. That is much to do in the matter of time that I've got."

"Well, we thought it to be prudent to invite you to dinner. If you must go, then go." Joshua announced. She appeared to be saddened by the fact that she had to go.

"Are you sure you got to go Sis?"

"Umm…hello…yes Samone. I can't stand my own man up."

"You didn't have to do all that. I just asked a simple question and besides, I know you got to leave. I just wanted to show you in some way that I really didn't want you to go. That is all that was intended. Trust and believe."

"Oh, well you have a funny way of showing it. You could have chosen another selection of words to say." While speaking, she reached for her keys in her purse. Once she retrieved them, she stood.

"I just want to say I do appreciate the gesture of inviting me to dinner, but unfortunately, I do have to go. We will definitely have to pick this up at a later date." We both stood.

She exited the booth and so did I. We hugged and she promised to call me later. She gave Joshua a slight hug, waved at us both, and exited the building. She was gone. My sister was gone. I was hurt for a moment, but it passed as the waitress came back with our drinks. She noticed that one of our parties was gone, but she didn't say anything. Kimberley just put Dedra's water back unto her tray.

To make sure she wasn't making a mistake, she asked, "You won't need this drink, will you?"

"No," I said.

I was very glad that the uniforms included the waiters and waitresses' names, so the consumers had an idea of whom to blame if something went wrong.

"Kimberley, we are both ready to order now."

"Alright Sir. What would you like?"

"I would like to have the baby back ribs dinner, with mash potatoes and corn as the side dishes." Kimberley had her order book in hand and was taking down the order as he spoke.

"Anything else Sir?"

"No, that's it for me."

"…and for you, Ma'am?" Just as I was about to speak, Joshua took the liberty to speak for me.

"Oh, my wife here will have the…umm, let me guess…"

He looked at me with a smirk on his face. He knew that I would get a kick out of the use of the word wife.

"…the buffalo wings with blue cheese and fries."

I was very impressed, for that was what I was going to order. I looked at him and then her with amazement in my eyes. Kimberley looked at our hands and realized that we weren't married, at least to the natural eye. Kimberley looked at me to make sure that that was what I wanted.

"Oh, um, yes. That's fine."

With a smile, she took the menus from us and said, "Your orders will be right out. Would you like any appetizers?"

"Um…as a matter of fact, I would. I would like your nacho cheese dip and chips." I looked from Kimberley's face to Joshua to see if he was happy with the selection I made.

"Yeah, that sounds good."

"Alright, I'll have that out to you really quick."

"Thanks…Miss."

"Her name is Kimberley Baby."

He looked from me to her and stated, "Oh, thanks Kimberley." She gave me a royal grin as to thank me for noticing her name.

Kimberley looked to be around my age and she had rosy cheeks that flickered her smile all the more. Her eyes were blue, she had brown hair, and her long slender legs made her look to be around 5'9 inches. She was pretty and very friendly. I like her perkiness and interest in her job. She left the table to go and retrieve our nacho cheese dip and chips.

"I bet she likes being a waitress," I said.

"Nah, I think she just do because she couldn't find anything else right now."

"Do we have a bet?" He looked at me with passion in his eyes. Joshua loved competition and bets.

"Now, you know we got a bet."

I sipped some of my water and asked him, "What were you two talking about when I was on the phone with my mother?"

"Oh, nothing really. She was just telling me about her new boyfriend." He looked around to examine the room to make sure no one was listening to our conversation.

"Really? You mean to tell me she told you about him before she told me anything. How could she? I was the first to ask her anyway."

"I don't know, Sweetheart that's just the way the cookie crumbled this time."

"The cookie crumble? What?" I knew he was just being silly, for he grabbed my hand and kissed it.

"So, now you have information about my sister that is vital, do you care to share or what?"

"Ok…ok…she said his name is Brian Johnson and he works for the District Attorney's office. He is a fine lawyer. She told me that he has actually heard of me through some friends of his down at the Austin Police Department. I have heard of him because he is pretty good at what he does and he has made his name well known. Most crooks he has been able to get off the street, but he hasn't been so successful with me. My lawyer is good at what he does too, that's why I pay him the big bucks. When I told her that I heard of him too, she shied from speaking more about him because she knew we were basically enemies. I tried to get more information out of her, but she just left it at he is a lawyer."

Marveled at what she just told me, I thought to myself, *"my big sister got herself a lawyer."*

At first, I couldn't believe it, but it sunk in and I realized that it was true. Joshua had no reason to lie about him. My sister has so many good things going on in her life. I can't be anymore happier for her than I already am.

"A lawyer, huh? That's really great for her. She deserves it."

"Are you trying to imply something?"

"What are you talking about," I asked? By this time, the waitress made it back with our chips and nacho dip.

"Is there anything else I can get you?"

"No. Not right now," Joshua shooed her away.

Kimberley just smiled and walked away with nothing else said.

"Never mind, I'm just going to leave it at that, I don't feel like getting into a heated discussion."

"A heated discussion? Why would it end up being a heated discussion?"

"I said never mind, Samone just leave it alone."

I took a chip in my hand and put some dip on it. As it entered my mouth, I could feel the steam rising to the roof of my mouth; once it hit my tongue, I was in Heaven. The cheese was a delight to chew. It had the taste of tomatoes, onion, and seasoned ground beef. From the moment I ate that first chip, I knew I could eat the whole thing.

"You better dig in while it's hot Joshua." He smacked his lip and gave me an attitude.

"What's wrong? Why are you acting so grumpy?"

"I'm not acting grumpy. I'm acting regular."

"I know you are not tripping about what I had to say about my sister, are you?" He looked at me, pissed.

"And what if I am? What are you going to do?"

"I knew it. I just don't understand why. I mean, all I said is that she has herself a lawyer and that she deserves it. What is so bad about that?"

He couldn't say anything, so he just sat there and watched me eat. I wasn't going to let Joshua ruin my dinner because of his insecurities about his profession. He could be pissed all he wanted to; I didn't care.

"It's just I know that you want me to get a legitimate job and I won't right now. It makes me jealous as hell when I think about you thinking of another man having a good job. Call me weird if you want to, but that's how I feel," he said with a softer tone.

I could tell that he had calmed down and wanted to talk things over like two grown adults.

"Well, I'm sorry you feel that way because I wasn't thinking that at all. I was just congratulating my sister to you instead of her because she isn't here." He picked up a chip and began to explore his taste buds with the scrumptious dip.

"Hmm, this is good, huh? That's why your butt over there eating it all up." He let out a little laugh as to break the ice that he made.

I just looked at him. "Yep, it is good."

Kimberley came back with our dinners. When she placed Joshua's plate down in front of him, I took a look at his food. I could tell that it was hot, for I seen the steam rise above from his plate. His food looked so good it made me envy his selection. After looking at his, I looked down at mine and I can honestly say, that it smelled like it was hot and it made my mouth water. After tasting both entrées, I must admit they were both delicious, for Joshua's food was meaty, tender, and rich with flavor; mine, on the other hand, was spicy, juicy, and mouthwatering.

"Do you like your food?" I asked.

He didn't take his eyes off his plate while he answered me, "Sure, it's alright."

"Joshua stop playing around. I know you know that the food tonight is very good. I can tell by the way you are gulping it down instead of swallowing." He finished his food and grabbed one of my wings.

"I should have ordered what you got," he said while chewing.

"That is something we both have in common; I was thinking the same thing about your food."

"You liked my ribs that much?"

"Yes. And you did too."

"How are you going to tell me what I enjoyed the most? I just said I should have ordered what you got, meaning that I didn't think my meal was good as yours. I ate all my food because I was hungry and I didn't want to waste my money."

"Why didn't you speak up then? We could have switched plates."

"I didn't know you liked my ribs."

"You know what...let's just end this conversation. It's senseless."

He exhaled, "You know what you are right. It is senseless. Who cares, right?"

"Right."

"So, why don't you hurry up so I can take you on home and by the way, I can't stay over tonight."

"Don't rush me and why aren't you staying over tonight?"

"Oh, I got to go and see my probation officer in the morning again."

"You sure have been going to see him enough lately. Why all the sudden meetings?"

"Do I sense attitude in the air?"

"No, just curiosity."

"Well, for your information, my parole officer is a female and she wants to discuss my job situation. She wants to make sure I'm not selling anymore…"

"But you are." I cut in.

"…what? No, I'm not selling. I have others who are selling it for me, but really that is on hold right now." He looked at me in this bizarre kind of way that it made me shiver.

"Why are you looking at me like that? Please stop, you are making me shiver." At first, he didn't respond to my request; he just stared at me.

"I'm just amazed at how I'm telling you all my business. I mean, business nobody knows but Tyrone. It makes me feel kind of weird." I felt very exceptional to the gesture of him trusting and believing in me to keep his secrets.

"I'm really glad that you are this open with me because I know most men in your predicament would not tell their woman anything. They would keep everything discreet and on the down-low," I grabbed his hand in mine and made eye contact, "so, thanks Baby. Thanks for believing in me." He smiled and told me that there was no need to thank him.

"I hope Tyrone is not telling Michelle any of my business, I know they are really tight; they are like Bonnie and Clyde. Just the other day, Michelle was asking me for some work to do. She gets a real kick out of the thug life. I don't mean to talk about your friend, but she is a little twisted. That's why deep inside, I knew they were meant for each other."

Joshua knew exactly how to change a subject that he did not care to talk about. He knew I had other questions about his "parole officer," but I was too enthused by what he was saying about Michelle. It made me realize the type of woman she really was and the kind of woman who could have my life in her hands, instead of the other way around. It made me look at her from a different light. Maybe all the crying she did was just to make me think that she wasn't involved with the whole thing that happened earlier today. Maybe she and Tyrone were in on it together. The question now is, what was it for? What are they trying to gain? I remember Michelle telling me one day that she wished that Tyrone were in the position that Joshua was in, making all the calls and calling the shots, that is. I remember thinking to myself; she must be crazy. What woman would want their man to be selling dangerous drugs to human life and feel no guilt? I remember asking Joshua if he felt guilty about selling to people and knowing what it does to them.

He answered, "At first I did but now it is so routine that I'm used to it. Baby, I'm just making money; that's all."

I remembered looking at him with disgust. I didn't make things better because I was in love with him. I just hope that the cops or other drug lords don't come after me because of him. Sad to say, I think two are already after me because of him.

"What are you thinking about Samone?" He shook my hand to get my attention, "what are you thinking about because you are in deep thought?"

"Oh, I was just thinking about what you were saying about Michelle."

"Ok…what about it because you had this distant look within your eyes. I know you were thinking more than what you are saying," he looked at me with concerned eyes, "you can tell me Sweetheart. I know there is something wrong with you because you have been distant ever since this morning. What really happened today?" I felt that Michelle was lying about something; I just can't put my finger on it.

"Samone, you can tell me anything. I tell you everything about my life and you know it's hard for me to open up to you about things. We promised that we wouldn't keep secrets from each other. So, tell me."

A flashback of the gun being shown to me with threats of using it crossed my mind, "You better not tell anyone about this."

I didn't know if I should tell him or still keep it secret. I was caught in between life and death. I started to think about the whole incident again, but wouldn't let my mind drift that far off, for Joshua was just staring at me waiting for my answer.

"The hell with it. I just hope nobody dies."

"WHAT! Die! What are you talking about?" Joshua almost yelled, "who is going to die? Who said something to you about dying? Speak up Samone, tell me." Tears began to flow from my eyes like a river.

Joshua stood up and put 60 dollars on the table which was more than enough.

"Come on, let's go. We have to finish this discussion in private." He took me by the hand and led me to the door.

Soon as we sat down in the car at Chili's parking lot, I let out the secret that was eating at me inside, "This morning...I didn't blackout or go into one of my episodes. I lied about the whole situation because I was told I better not tell anyone. Michelle and I were at the house and I remember her ordering a pizza because we both didn't want to cook."

"Damn the pizza. Just get to the part about dying."

"Hold on, Joshua let me tell the story. Anyway, 15 minutes later, Tyrone knocked on the door and I let him in, I think, I'm not sure, maybe it was Michelle."

"I don't care who let him in. I will kill that fool if he hurt you." He started the car and began to ease his foot off the brakes.

"Where are we going?"

"I am going over Tyrone's house to finish this."

"Nooo, don't do that. I swear if you do, I will jump out of this car. I am not even playing."

"Aw, so that fool did do something to you? You don't even want to face him. What did he say to you? Damn it, Samone spit it out. What did that bastard say to you?"

"If you would only let me speak, maybe I could get it out. As I was saying, Tyrone began to spit out that he was tired of "friends" interfering with his relationships. He said that he didn't like the idea of me telling Michelle that they should wait on getting married. Then the next thing I know he was in my face. By this time, I was already nervous because he was yelling. Michelle tried to calm him down, but it didn't work. He called me ugly and told me to stay out of their business or else. He motioned for me to look down and I saw his gun. I asked him what he was planning to do with his gun and he told me that I was going to find out if I stayed in their business."

My face was wet with tears and I was actually surprised that he understood everything that came out of my mouth, for I was sobbing so much.

"He said if I told anyone that he was going to kill Michelle and me. He told me not to even tell you. I wasn't going to tell you at first because I know you have a hot temper and things would explode but…" Joshua took me in his arms and tried to calm me down.

"Calm down Baby… it's ok. I'm going to take care of everything." Joshua said in a surprisingly calm voice.

"What are you going to do Joshua? I don't want anyone to die or get hurt."

"Samone, I want you to know that I'm glad that you came correct with telling the truth. That is some information that I truly needed to know. I can't believe that you were actually considering keeping that secret from me. I would have been upset with you if you would have waited longer to tell me." He kissed me on the lips.

"I love you and I am going to take care of everything. You don't have to worry about a thing. Your life is in good hands. I know people, Samone. Maybe I shouldn't be telling you this, but I am I know killers. I know men who owe me favors and would not hesitate doing it. I can't believe that Tyrone would do something like this, though."

"Baby, don't kill nobody. You should have kept that to yourself. I don't want to be the blame for anyone dying." There was silence the whole way home. He put the car in park and turned to face me.

"Samone, Baby, I'm sorry that you had to go through what you went through, but trust me, things will be better for you, don't worry one bit." He kissed me on the forehead, nose, and then my lips.

"I want you to stay with me tonight."

"I know you do, but I can't, I got to take care of some things. Besides, I wouldn't be able to comfort you too much because I have so many emotions and thoughts going on in my head."

"What do you think I'm going through? I know about that, remember my condition?"

"Damn…Baby, I'm sorry, but I got to go." I jumped out of the car and slammed the door.

I yelled at him, "I can't believe out of all the nights I need you; you won't stay. How can you say you love me? You don't love me." He got out of the car and tried to console me, but I wouldn't let him touch me.

"Ok…it's like that Samone? You don't want me to touch you…okay, it's cool. I'll just stand here until you go inside."

"Well, I got the mind to stay out here all night just to make sure you are here with me."

"Samone, damn Woman, would you just let me go? I have somewhere to be that has to do with business, don't take this shit so personal, damn."

"Oh yeah, where do you have to be? Is it your parole officer's place?"

"See, your ass is tripping now. First of all, I'm not loving anybody but your ass. Second, she is my parole officer and nothing else. Third, it's late and I'm trying to take care of your ass and mine at the same time. I can't believe that you would think that I would cheat on you. I have somewhere to be Woman and that's that. Now take your ass in the house and lock up and I will call you when I'm done."

"Joshua, if you go to prison, I'm not waiting for you, I hope you know that. You said you were not doing anything illegal right now."

"I know what I told you. I said that I have people doing it for me. That's what I said."

"Well, why do you have to go then? You know what…goodnight." I turned my back to him and started walking toward my apartment.

I heard him yell after me, "I'm gonna call you and I love you!"

I turned around and yelled back at him, "Don't even bother!"

He got me so upset that I didn't want to hear his voice or see him. I just wanted to be left alone by him. I opened the door and through my purse and cell phone on the couch. Soon as I sat my stuff down, my cell phone rang. I sat down while I looked to see who the caller was and it was Joshua. I just looked at the phone while it rang. I wasn't about to answer that phone, he made me upset, so he didn't deserve to hear my voice. I got up from the couch and went into the bathroom to take my medicine.

"Who does Joshua think he is?" I thought to myself.

I mean, he knows about Tyrone and he just left me here all by myself because he "has to take care of some business." He could have made a rain check on that. I'm more important than his job. At least I think so. Maybe I'm not. I got tired of hearing that phone rang, so I went back to pick up the phone once I swallowed my pill. It was an intermission between calls and I was able to see how many times he called. The phone indicated five times. Just when I was about to sit the phone down, it rang, but it wasn't Joshua; it was Michelle. She must be calling me to check up on me and to see how dinner went. I hope she is not the woman Joshua described to me because I'm in way over my head if she is.

"Hello," I said.

"So, how was dinner?" Michelle sounded so dry and shaky with her question. It almost seemed as if she was being forced to ask the question.

"Dinner was good. You should have come along with us."

"Oh, I was, but there was some unfinished business I had to take care of. You can understand that, right?"

"Yeah, I understand."

"So, where is your boyfriend? Is he there with you?"

For some reason, something in me told me to lie to her, I didn't trust her knowing that I was home alone, so I did.

"Yeah, he's here. He's in the bathroom."

"Oh, well, while both of you are still there, maybe me and Tyrone can come over and hang out."

"Nah, I don't think that is a good idea; we are getting ready for bed. You know how that is."

"Oh, ok. Well, maybe some other time. Samone, you didn't snitch, did you?"

"No."

"Are you sure…because if you did and I find out you are lying to me….I'm going to…well, let's just say that it wouldn't be good for you to be lying right now."

"Michelle, I don't have to lie to you. I didn't say a word to him about what happened. Besides, he still thinks I had one of my episodes."

"Well, I hope so, for your sake."

"And what does that supposed to mean, Michelle?"

"It means what it sounds like."

"Michelle, are you making threats at me? What is going on with you? You seem like you are changing into this person that I never knew. You are supposed to be my sister and here you are making a threat on my life. How could you?"

"Well, I'm sorry you feel that way, but I have to make sure you don't tell a soul what happened because my life is on the line too. I mean, if you go and tell Joshua what happen there is going to be a war between the two of them; that is what I'm trying to stop. I don't want that little incident to interfere with what we got going on now. I talked to Tyrone about the situation and he regrets even doing that to you. I know you may not believe it, but he is really sorry for what he did. Can you just find it in your heart to forgive him?"

"What!?! Are you serious? He is nothing more than a dangerous villain out there in the streets. If I were you, I would leave him. You say your life is in danger too, well, why stay with him? And by your threats on my life leads me to believe that you are willing to do whatever it takes to keep him happy. Girl, can't you see he is playing you?"

"Be careful about what you say about my man. I don't say anything negative about yours, so keep all the drama to yourself."

She paused for a moment and mumbled under her breath, "I can't take this pretending anymore."

"What did you say Michelle? You can't take what pretending anymore?"

"If you heard what I said, why ask me to repeat it?"

"Umm, helloo to make sure what I heard was accurate, that's why."

I could tell I was beginning to piss her off. I could feel the steam getting hotter and hotter off the phone and maybe some of that steam was some of mine as well.

"You better watch your tone with me Samone. I'm not the one to play with."

"Do you think I should have a reason to fear you? You are only human, just like I am. You bleed, I bleed, we both bleed. Do you get the point?"

She started to laugh an evil laugh, and she said, "Are we growing some balls or what? You keep surprising me Samone, you really do. I can't believe you are trying to intimidate me over the phone. I mean, that is something I wouldn't in a hundred years imagine you to do. But now on a serious tip…you should have a reason to fear me. Let's just say, I have done some dirty work for Tyrone and I don't regret or feel anything about it." Silence was in the air; it was so strong I could smell it, taste it, heck, I could see the silence.

"Oh, so we have nothing to say? You not talking shit now, what's up?"

"Look, I don't care what you may have did for Tyrone. That shit is done and over with, we are talking about here and now."

"Samone…do you really think you can take me on?"

"Look, Michelle, my life is nothing to play with. Why don't you take your threats and ideas about death somewhere else? I can deal without them."

"Nah, I want to settle this. I want you to back all your bravery up. You are talking lots of mess and I want to see what you can do."

"So, what are you purposing? You want us to meet up somewhere like schoolgirls and duke it out?"

"Nah, nothing like that. I just want you to be ready for what is about to happen to you." With that, she hung up the phone and left me without anything to say.

I didn't know what she meant or how she was going to do it; all I know is that she was planning my death. Now, what was I going to do? I didn't have a gun; to be honest, I hated guns. Joshua knew all along that she was crazy. The woman just told me, in so many words, that she killed someone. I couldn't believe that Michelle would do such a thing. She put on a good impersonation. She really only allowed me to see what she wanted me to see. We were made believe sisters to the heart and now all that was disappearing. We had just begun to be enemies and to tell you the truth, I preferred being made believe sisters. There was something about Michelle that just wasn't right. Like Joshua, I just couldn't put my finger on it. Besides the fact that she was a complete lunatic, she scared me a little. The way she was talking to me over the phone made me shiver. She spoke with a spooky nonchalant voice. I believe I asked for trouble with my words. Maybe I shouldn't have acted so big and bad over the phone, I mean, I don't have any weapons to back me up. However, I bet Michelle has all types of guns in her collection. I bet she has every one of them named and categorized into sections. I wonder how many guns she had for that matter. I can't believe what I just did. I put my life in more danger than it already was; I have to change the situation someway. I took the phone in my hand and began to dial Joshua's number. Hopefully, he wasn't upset with me for not answering his phone calls, for I needed to talk with him. On the second ring, he answered the phone.

"Oh, so now you want to talk with me. What took you so long? Are you still angry with me?"

"Well, to be honest, yes, I'm still angry with you, but I have to tell you what just happened. Michelle and I shared some words and now she wants to do harm to me."

"What!?! What was said Samone?"

"I basically told her that I didn't care that she handled some of Tyrone's dirty work. She told me that she didn't feel any regrets about doing it either. Joshua, the woman just told me that she killed someone. She also said that I should keep a lookout on what is going to happen to me."

"Damn Samone, it's enough that I have to worry about Tyrone, now I have to worry about his damn crazy woman too. This is too much." He paused before he kept going. "…I was trying to call you and let you know what's up with Tyrone. The word on the street is he wants my spot. He wants to call all the shots. He has been a busy little bee. Tyrone has been trying to recruit some of my very own men behind my back. I don't know what's his problem is, he should know my men are loyal to me and they are going to let me know what's up. I've been trying to call him and see what's up with him, but he won't answer my calls. I even got desperate enough to call Michelle; she answered and said that she didn't know where he was. She was lying; she knew where he was. He was probably there listening to us conversing."

"Joshua, I don't know what to do. I don't know what they are capable of."

"Um, hello…Samone, can you say murder?"

"What should I do?"

"Well, right now I'm in the middle of something, but I'm going to be there soon. Ooh, I got an idea. Maybe you can call your mom or your sister to come and get you if you don't feel safe there by yourself."

"Hell no, I don't feel safe. I'm on the lookout for my life Joshua and you are too. You better believe Tyrone is going to be coming after you."

"Yeah, I know. You are so right."

"Joshua, remember when I told you that I didn't want to be caught up in the middle or basically, to be used to get to you?"

"Yeah, I remember that and I know what you are going to say. Tyrone and Michelle are using you to get to me. Don't worry, Samone I know what I am doing, even if I have to go to jail to protect you, I will."

"That's the thing; I don't want you to go to jail. Just give in and let Tyrone have the business. Joshua, just get out the game."

"Woman, have you taken your medicine? I can't do that shit; I'm too deep in it. I got to handle this like I would anything else."

"Do you know what you are doing?"

"No, not really. My main supporter has gone astray and he can't come back. His deranged and lunatic woman is no better. I think she is the one that put all this "taking over Joshua's loot" into his head. I can't believe that it worked because he and I were super tight. I mean, I just can't believe it." I didn't want to make him feel any worse by telling him I told you so, so I just sat on the phone and listened.

"Samone, I'm going to need you. I'm going to need you to make some moves for me. If you want to survive this, you are going to have to get gangsta' on Michelle."

"So, what are you saying? I'm going to have to kill her? I don't do murders Joshua. I just don't do that."

"God no, I didn't mean that. What I mean is, I'm going to need you to outsmart her. You got a brain Samone, use it. You be thinking of all kinds of things, you can set her up some kind of way."

The man was right; I could come up with something to get her ass in trouble with the law. All I had to do was search around for some truth and get her.

"You are right Joshua. There is something I can do without pulling a trigger, but for right now I need you to come over here and be with me. Is there anyone that you can trust that can finish the job that you are doing right now?"

"Well, actually, I'm almost done and I should be over there shortly. I would much rather you go over your mother's or sister's house."

"Ok…Joshua, I will give Dedra a call."

He sighed with relief, "Thank you so much for doing that. Now I can finish this with more ease."

"Um Joshua, just because I call them doesn't mean they will come and get me."

"Woman please, you know your mama is overprotective of you two. She would drop whatever it is she is doing to come and rescue you and you know that."

I must admit the man knew my mother, even though they didn't get along, he knew her well. I sat on the phone in silence. Now that I heard his voice, I didn't want to get off the phone with him. Hearing his reassurance that my life will be spared made me feel safe and secure even though he wasn't at the house with me.

"Samone, are you there?"

"Oh, um, yeah, I'm here. I just don't want to get off the phone with you. You are really making me feel safe right now."

"I'm glad I can do that for you, but unfortunately, I must go. I know you don't want me to, but I have to."

"Ok…I'm going to call Dedra now."

"Good. Call me back to let me know what she is going to do."

"Ok."

"I love you very much Samone and I'm doing everything in my power to make sure you stay from any harm."

I smiled, "I love you too. Bye for now."

"Bye, for now." I hung up the phone and dialed my sister's phone number. On the fourth ring, she answered the phone.

"Hello."

"Hey Sis, are you busy?"

"Um…sort of, why?" I had a feeling she was with Brian, but I settled not to say so.

"Well, I was wondering if you could come and get me."

"Come and get you…," she echoed, "…why do I need to come and get you?"

"Well, it's a long story, but just know this, I may be in danger."

"What are you talking about Samone? What danger? I mean, are you playing a joke on me or what? I'm trying to get some sleep and…"

"Hold on…wait a minute Dee. I'm serious as a heart attack. Some stuff went down and I got to get away from my apartment for a while."

"Does this have anything to do with that boyfriend of yours?"

"Can you come and get me or what?"

"Well, I'm with Brian right now, but I'm sure he will understand. I'll be over there within an hour. I'm not coming in, so listen for my horn."

"Ok. Bye."

I heard her exhale and she then replied, "Bye."

I knew she really didn't want to travel the distance over here, for I heard it all in her voice, but she was and that is what counts. For the most part, I can depend on my sister for just about anything and I am happy about that because many people won't do the things my sister and I do for one another. I began to prepare a night bag for my stay. I grabbed some clothes, shoes, undergarments, and my medicine. I didn't know how long I would be over my sister's house, so I just packed enough clothing to last me throughout the whole week.

There was a knock on the door. I knew it couldn't be my sister, for she lives pretty far from where I live.

I walked to the door, "Who is it?" I asked.

"Open the door, Samone it's me."

"Me who?"

"Oh, so you don't know my voice now?"

Only one person complained about everything I did, so I knew exactly who it was. I opened the door and he walked into my apartment.

"Girl, I thought you weren't gonna' open the door there for a minute. Next time I need you to open the door more quickly." I looked at him in a problematic way.

"Charles, what are you doing here so late? You know my man would have a field day if he were here."

"Yeah, I know, but he is not here and I knew he wouldn't be here."

Love's Mirage

"How did you know that?" I asked.

He smiled, "Samone...Samone... now you know I can't give out that kind of information."

"Why not? I can keep a secret." Charles made his way to my couch and sat down.

"Um, who told you to get comfortable? I'm about to leave in a few minutes. You got to make your way out of this house."

"You sure you want me to go? Word on the street is someone doesn't like you and they wouldn't mind seeing you dead." I stood there with my mouth open.

I was amazed at how this man could go months without speaking or seeing me and know exactly what was going on in my life. I mean, he knew personal things. I'm surprised he didn't know about my diagnosis. I slowly sat down to face him.

"Charles..."

He put his hand up, grabbed my hand in his and said, "Woman, we could leave right now. I got the means to take care of you. I know you are scared and I want to comfort you. I don't know if you know this already, but someone has put a hit out on Joshua too. Samone, Baby, you need to get away from here. Let me take care of you."

He stood up to pull something from his pants. It was a document that was addressed to me.

"Look, I'm not here to judge you or make fun of you but, you really need to up your game because that girl Michelle put this on my car." He handed me the paper and it read: Hey fool, that bitch that you claim you in love with is dead. Signed someone who hates you too.

After reading the note, I looked at Charles.

All I could say was, "What?" He shrugged his shoulders as if he knew exactly what I was trying to say.

"I don't know Samone. As soon as I got that letter, I hurried over here to make sure you were okay."

"Where were you? I mean, she must have just placed this on your car."

"Why do you say that?"

"Because me and her just got off the phone earlier this evening. It hasn't been that long since I have talked with her."

"Well, she caught me while I was at work."

"How does she know where you work?"

He looked at me, surprised and said, "I don't know; maybe you told her." I began to backtrack to see if I did spill the goods on where he worked and couldn't remember doing so.

"No, I didn't tell her anything."

"Well, I don't know how she figured out where I work. But damn all that, what are you going to do? Are you going to stay here and wait to see if she really mean what she say? Or are you going to take a ride with me? And if you choose to stay here, you really got to be prepared. You can't fight bullets Samone." I looked down at the letter again and shook my head.

"I don't know what I want to do Charles. I mean, if I go with you, I will be running and I would probably have to do that for the rest of my life."

"I know you would be safe wit' me. I don't got no beef with anyone."

Just when I thought Charles had changed his English, the slang once again entered into his mouth, but at this point, I didn't care. All that mattered was that someone was with me that cared about me. I got up from my seat and sat down beside Charles.

"Thanks for coming to check on me, even though you could have caused me drama if my man were here, but then again, you knew that he wasn't here. So, tell me, would you have done the same thing even if you knew that Joshua was here?"

He looked into my eyes and said, "Hell yeah, I would've did the same thang. I don't care about Joshua; Samone. He is not good for you like I am. First of all, I wouldn't put you in no bad situation that could cost you your life, like he did..." He stood up and began to pace the floor gradually. "...puttin' you in the middle of this shit, who do he think he is? Second of all, he not even here with you right now and he should be. Third of all, guess who is here with you right now? Someone who loves your ass." He spoke out loud so that I could hear his thoughts, but he wasn't speaking directly to me.

He turned his attention back to me. "Let me take care of you Samone. You won't have to want for nothing."

"Charles you are putting me in an awkward situation. There is a part of me that is saying go with Charles, but then the majority of me is saying stay right here and finish this." Charles walked over to me and got on his knee. I shied.

"Charles, what are you doing?" He looked as if I disappointed him by asking him what he was doing.

So with reluctance, he said, "Don't worry...Samone, I wasn't fixin' to ask you to marry me, even though I had thoughts about asking you. All I know is you would probably end up sayin' no. And that would hurt my heart, just like you are doing right now. All you have to do is come with me. That's all." His voice began to crack as if he were about to let loose tears.

I looked at him with concern in my eyes. Deep inside, something told me that this man would love me and all I had to do was step out on a limb. Then there was the other part of me that said I must stay. I was so confused; I didn't know what to do. He looked at me with tears in his eyes and then looked away. I put my hand on his chin to turn his face to face mine again. I kissed him and then he kissed back. He got up from his knees which caused me to stand up with him. I had my arms around his broad shoulders and he had my size seven waist in his hands. We were going at when all of a sudden, I noticed a piece of paper under my door.

I pulled away, "Wait a minute."

"What's going on Samone?" I walked over to find out what the letter was about.

And it read, "I know you don't know me, but I found out some information that may interest you. Please call me as soon as possible. (512)555-9563. Sincerely, Call me to see.

I took the note and threw it out of frustration.

"What in the hell is going on Charles?" He picked the letter up and began to read it. He looked at me and shook his head.

"I don't know what to tell you Samone. You really do need me to take you away from here."

"I told you Charles, I can't run away from this. It is just going to follow me wherever I go." Charles walked over to me and hugged me.

"I know you still love me; you wouldn't have given me that kiss if you didn't. Just let me return the favor unto you by loving you."

"I…I…can't do that. Not just yet. Charles, I do still love you, but things are not going good right now. It wouldn't be prudent for us to start something right now."

"See, that's where we are dif'rent...my bad different. I think any time to be with you is a good time."

This man was very persistent; I had to give him that. And everyone knew that being persistent with me usually got the seeker what they wanted. I exhaled.

"What's wrong?"

"I got too much stress right now. That's what's wrong with me." He looked down at the letter in his hand again.

"Are you going to call this number?"

"Not right now Charles. My sister is on her way and I need to be getting ready for her arrival."

"Is that a sign for me to leave?"

"Take it the way you want to Charles."

He smacked his lips; ugh, you don't have to get nasty with me Samone. I'm the man here wanting to take you away from all this stress. I'm the man who wanna' love you like you never been loved. Treat me wit' some respect."

"I will when you learn how to talk."

"What's that?"

"His feelings were hurt."

"When I what? Look, I know you are under some stress, so Imma leave you alone bout' that. But know this, I'm not gonna wait too long."

With that, he pulled out his keys and left my apartment, which made me feel lousy. I couldn't believe I said that out loud. I was only thinking it. I didn't expect it to come out as it did. I hurt his feelings and I knew I did for he left me alone. I deserved what he did to me. I mean, the man was just exposing his love for me and I just spat it back in his face. The man wanted to take me away and what did I do? I turned him down because of Joshua. I felt very foolish. Fooling around with Joshua may cost me my life, but Charles wanted to take me somewhere and give me a life.

"How stupid can you be Samone?" I said to myself. Then I remembered the letter, *"Did Charles take it with him?"* I thought to myself. I looked around for it and I couldn't find it. He took it with him. That's how he is aware of what is going on with me. He purposely takes all vital information on me and investigates it independently. It wouldn't surprise me if he knew about my diagnosis. Now I am going to have to call him to get that number. By the time I do, he will probably be able to tell me what the person got to say. Exhausted by all the stress, I sat down on the couch to relax until my sister made it. It wasn't long till she came either, for I was able to relax only 30 minutes. Then she pulled up and honked the horn.

CHAPTER FIVE

I grabbed my keys, bag, purse, and cell phone and headed toward the door. When I locked my door, I turned around to see that my sister was facing me. I let out a surprised scream.

"I thought you weren't going to get out of the car?"

"Well, I wouldn't have if I didn't have to honk my horn so many times. What took you so long? Are you alright?" I followed her back to her running car and got into the passenger's seat.

"...to answer your questions, no, I'm not alright. And I had to look for my keys. Girl, there is so much stuff going on in my life that I don't know where to begin." She looked at me while backing out the parking space and then turned her attention back to driving.

"Well, just start anywhere that you feel you are comfortable enough to talk about. It must be something big for you to ask me to come and get you in the middle of the night. You better be glad that you are my sister and I love you very much because if you wasn't..." I began to tune out her explanation of her reason of coming over to get me.

"Dedra." I haven't called her by her name in a long time, so when I did it shocked her.

"You know what, I can't remember the last time you called me by my name. What's going on Samone?"

"Well, you know Michelle, right?"

"Yeah. Of course."

"Well, she got beef with me and now she has declared that she is going to take my life."

"What!?!" my sister said in disbelief, "what happened Samone? I mean, are you sure this is the same Michelle that we have known since school? What is wrong with her? Why is she tripping? Is she really capable of doing something like that?"

"Now that's the million-dollar question. That's what you should have been asking all along. And the answer is yes."

"How do you know?" We were on I-35 when I noticed an accident.

"Sis, we are in for a wait. Look." I pointed my index finger toward the accident.

"Great. How am I going to get rest now? I got to work tomorrow. But anyway, back to the question I asked you. How do you know?"

"She told me that she did some dirty work for Tyrone and that she didn't have any regrets about doing it."

"For real? I can't believe that Michelle would do something like that. That's just not her character."

"Believe it. Joshua tried to warn me about her in his own way. He use to always say… "I don't know about that girl. Something ain't right about her." I would blow him off and just think he was joking around because you know Michelle is silly, but sure enough, he ended up being right."

"You need to really call the police, Samone. We will call them we get to my place. They need to be involved so they can protect your life."

"I can't do that Dedra."

"And why not?" I could hear the dismissal in her tone.

"Because. I have to take care of this myself."

We began to slow down; traffic policeman was directing us. The accident was a horrific scene. One of the cars was flipped upside down. There were ambulances, fire trucks, police cars, and state troopers parked around the other vehicle. Channel 7 News was also there. That was the station Michelle's sister worked for. I wouldn't be surprised to see her there. From what I was able to see, there were a couple of bodies on stretchers. They were covered in blood.

"Oh, my goodness. I hope they are alright," I said.

I was able to catch a glimpse of what happened and that was it. Unexpectedly, the traffic was moving along, even though there were still those nosey onlookers.

"I don't know why every time there is a traffic accident; it has to be so slow. All the drivers have to do is keep going. Someone have to always be nosey to see what is going on. Damn people, they are making me sick."

"Calm down Sis…we will get through this soon."

"Anyway, back to what I asked you. Answer me."

"I did. I have to take care of this situation."

"Girl, are you crazy? You can't handle that crazy woman by yourself. Samone, listen to yourself. How can you take on someone who has experience in killing someone else? You can't. You just can't." Then she looked at me with curiosity.

"Are you trying to tell me something?"

"What…what do you mean?"

"Uh-huh Samone, tell me that you haven't killed someone before."

Out of all the things my sister has said to me over the years, this was by far the worst thing she has ever said to me.

"How in the world could you ever think I would or could do something like that? I can't believe you." I turned my back to her.

By me doing that I was able to tell her that I wasn't interested in conversing with her anymore.

"Samone…I'm sorry. I just don't know what to think or ask right now. My head has gone haywire from all this stuff that you are telling me. I can't believe that I truly thought that, let alone me actually saying it. Samone, I'm truly sorry."

Now I knew how Charles felt when I said what I said to him to hurt his feelings. She didn't know how much what she said affected me. Tears began to roll down my face.

With my back still facing her, I began to speak through my cries, "…and that's not even the whole story. There is plenty more from where that came from."

She was silent; she didn't say a word, which was very clever on her part. She knew if I wanted to talk, I would without her urging me. I turned around to face the dashboard.

"You really hurt my feelings, saying that type of rubbish. You should know I could never take anyone's life."

She still didn't say anything. I guess she was sulking. The car began to move at a decent speed.

"Seriously, what are you going to do about Michelle? To me, it seems like you are taking things so lightly like bad things won't happen. The truth of the matter is something bad could really happen to you. And I don't want to see nothing happen to you." Her voice cracked and I knew she was on the verge of tears.

"I do take this very seriously. I'm not taking any of this lightly. My life is in danger and I don't know which way to turn. It feels like I'm being backed up to a wall without any escape."

"Michelle. Samone, what are you going to do about her?" she asked in a calm voice.

Honestly, I was really getting tired of her asking about Michelle. The truth of the matter was, I didn't know. I didn't have the first clue as to what to do about her.

"I don't know, Sis. I really don't know."

She grabbed my hand and told me some comforting words. She told me that her lawyer boyfriend could maybe help. I refused that notion because that would only lead back to Joshua.

"Let Joshua take care of himself. You worry about you. Don't be foolish; let Brian help you. You wouldn't be in this mess if it wasn't for Joshua anyway. I told you he was no good and that it would end up this way."

I sat there and just listened to my sister. She was right. I wouldn't be in this mess if it weren't for Joshua. But a part of me couldn't give in. I love Joshua and I love Charles too. I wouldn't want anything bad to happen to either one of them.

"Sis, I got to tell you about Charles."

My sister met Charles one time when he dropped me off at her apartment and she enjoyed his company. He told some jokes, made us laugh, and even bought lunch. He impressed me at the time. I didn't know Charles had it in him to show some hospitality. My sister and Charles kept in touch over the last couple of months. He has even shared some of their conversations with me. Hmmpp, now that I think about it, my sister is another reason why he knows so much about me. She probably tells him and Brian everything about me. Yeah, I'm absolutely sure that he knows about my diagnosis. From what Charles told me, they are good friends. He told me that they hung out on a couple of occasions and he said they would always talk about me. He also told me that he would try to find out ways through Dedra to get my attention. She was never able to help in that field since I was so consumed with Joshua. He finished by telling me that my sister told him not to worry, that I would come around and love only him.

"How is Charles?" A smile came across her face diminishing her frown.

I must say something wasn't right about that. That smile made me feel uneasy and belittled. That piercing smile made me think something went on between the two of them.

"Charles, how could you?" I thought to myself.

"What about Charles? Is he alright? I haven't heard from him in a while." I was still thinking about that smile when she shook my shoulder.

"Samone, do you hear me talking to you?" I looked at her as she pulled into her reserved parking space outside of her townhouse apartment.

"Oh uh…yeah, I hear you. And yes, he is doing fine. He was over my house tonight before you made it over. He asked me if he could take me away from all of this."

"Really?" my sister said, surprised.

"Yes, really."

"That's good. Why don't you go with him? It seems like a great idea. He can take you away from all this mess and you won't have to worry about your life being in jeopardy."

We got out of the car and I started looking around to see if I could spot Brian's car, but I couldn't pinpoint his out. I followed my sister up the sidewalk to her apartment.

"I rejected his offer." I stopped my sister in the middle of her tracks.

"You what? Why would you do something like that? This is a man you so many times told me that you loved and adored. And you can't let him take you away? What's wrong with you?" she looked at me, disgusted and confused, "this is your perfect opportunity to getaway. Take it."

"Dedra, I don't know what to do. To be honest, a part of me wants to stay here and help Joshua and the other part wants to go with Charles. I'm so confused."

"What are you so confused about? You need to be going with Charles because Joshua is the one who got you in this mess in the first place. Why is it so hard for you to see that?"

"I feel like I can help Joshua out in some kind of way."

"Tell me, how can you help him? He is a grown man who makes his own decisions." She turned around and continued up the sidewalk, I followed.

"Honestly, Samone I don't know what's wrong with you."

I began to think about what my sister was telling me and I took every word into consideration for my final decision.

"Is Brian here?"

"I don't know. I told him I was going to pick you up and he told me that he might stay around and make sure everything was alright."

"You didn't tell him anything about me, did you?" Just as she was opening the door, she began to answer my question.

"I'm going to be honest with you. I told him some things about you. I didn't tell him everything, so don't worry."

"Oh my goodness...only God knows what this man I never met thinks of me. What did you tell him?"

"I told him that you have a dilemma in your present life. I didn't give him any details, but he already knew that you were Joshua's girlfriend when I mentioned your name to him."

"He what? How did he know me?"

"He knows who you are because he has been following up on Joshua Franks for some time now…"

"Well, just go on and spill all the beans out, Dedra, why don't you?"

I looked up to find a nice looking dark-skinned man standing in the hallway that led to the bedroom. Brian had a head full of deep natural black waves, a goatee that was cleverly designed, his shoulders were broad, and he stood about 5'11 inches. He walked over to where I was and stretched out his arm for me to shake his hand.

"Hello, I'm Brian. It's nice to finally meet the woman who is dating Joshua Franks." I gave my sister an awkward look. I reached out my hand and shook his.

"Hello, nice to meet you too. Since you already know who I am, there is really no need of me telling you who I am?" He smiled at me.

"So…" He looked at Dedra. "…what took you guys so long in getting here?" Dedra walked over to him and hugged him and he gave her a peck on the cheek.

"Oh, there was an accident." My sister's attitude had totally changed.

She went from being the person that I have known all my life, to this other woman. I mean, she was never an affectionate person. At least that is what she told me, but here she was given this man I did not know all the affection he wanted. I felt like a nosey onlooker. I really wasn't in the mood to see anybody smooch and show love.

"An accident, huh? Do you all know what happened?"

"No, we just pass by it on I-35." With my sister still in one of his arms, he turned his attention back to me.

"Did you see anything, Mrs. Franks?" He let out a laugh as he said it.

I gave him this dissatisfying look as to say I thought the remark wasn't funny.

"Now stop that, Brian don't do my sister that way."

I could already tell that I did not like this man. He was trying to be funny and it wasn't. The tone that he used led me to believe that he was trying to make me feel small because of my choice to date Joshua. He was ADA of Travis County, so I knew he didn't like Joshua and now I know he must not like me. He straightened up his composure and looked at me with curiosity in his eyes. I knew he wanted to ask me questions Joshua, for I was his key to success. With my help, he could capture Joshua. In my eyes, if I were him, I would try to get on my good side instead of the opposite. He was up to no good and I knew it.

"Why did I come here?" I thought to myself.

I exhaled and said, "Yes, I seen people covered with blood on stretchers."

"I apologize if I offended you in any way. Excuse my behavior."

I accepted his apology, but I was no fool. This man was out to get Joshua and probably me, who knows.

"Wow, I'm so sorry to hear that for those people. I hate when death comes around and take lives. It's a job that I wouldn't want to do."

"But Mr. Johnson, you do take lives. You put people behind bars for life and that in a way, is taking someone's life."

He looked at me with animosity as he contemplated the meaning of my words. My sister, on the other hand, had her mouth agape as the words ringed within her ears. I tried to hold it in, but I couldn't.

"That's what he gets for trying to make a fool of me."

Brian let out an uneasy laugh and said, "Well, you do have a point Samone, but you do realize that I meant physically taking someone's life, right?

I looked at him as if I were confused, and said, "Nah…do you think?" I could tell that I was making Brian frustrated by the wrinkles in his forehead.

"Ok, you two, this was not the first impression that I wanted you two to share. Let's just play this cool." Brian and I had locked eyes and were trying to stare the other down with resentment.

The air was hot-filled with heated emotions and the best idea my sister came up with to cool the situation down was to kiss Brian. It made me look away and it distracted him. I was tired of the whole confrontation anyway, so I just let it go. I don't think he did, for when they were done kissing, he gave me an evil glare. Dedra couldn't see the glare because they were hugging and her chin was on his shoulders.

"Well, ladies, I have to cut out of here. It was nice meeting you Samone and Dedra I'll give you a call when I make it to the house."

"Aw, why must you leave," my sister pleaded. She pulled his collar toward her to make him bend down to give her another kiss.

"Baby go ahead and be with you sister. I'll be back tomorrow."

Through the corner of my eyes, I could see that my sister was looking at me. I couldn't make out the expression on her face because I had my eyes on one of my most favorite pieces of artwork.

"Well, you take care and be sure to call me like you said."

"I will."

With that, he grabbed his keys from one of the end tables and headed toward the door; my sister followed. He opened it up and turned around to kiss my sister on the forehead.

"Take care of your sister."

"I will." She closed the door and turned her attention to me.

"You know all that kissing was disgusting to me."

"Why? Oh, I know, maybe it's because your life is not all the perfect right now."

She hurried and said, "Samone, why did you have to make those remarks?"

She didn't even give me a chance to respond to the last remark she made. I guess she intended it to be that way.

"What remarks?" I acted confused.

"You know what I'm talking about. You ran my man up out of here. He would have stayed if you hadn't made him upset."

"Hey, he said some words as well. Actually, he started it with all the laughing and Mrs. Franks jokes." I walked to the couch and sat down.

I looked down at the carpet as I said, "Dedra, I don't want to argue. I have had enough today." She walked over to where I was and sat down next to me.

"I don't want to argue either. I just wanted to know why you said the things you said; that's all. I mean, you shocked me with that taking the lives of criminals' remark."

"Well, I tried to hold it in, but I couldn't. It was lingering at the tip of my tongue burning to be said."

I looked at her in her eyes to show how sincere I was with my emotions and thoughts. I also grabbed her by the hand. I wanted to let her know that what I was about to say was from my heart and I meant it.

"Sis, I love you and I want nothing but the best for you. You know that, right?" I waited for an answer.

"Yeah. Why are you saying this?"

"Listen, Brian doesn't like me and I don't know if I like him, but as long as he makes you happy then I'll try to deal with him."

"Why don't you think he likes you?"

"Because…I just know he doesn't. What I get from Brian is…he is a man about his career. And his career has him after Joshua. He is going to try and get every little bit of information out of you about me and him." I took my face in my hands.

I exhaled through my hands and muffled some words, "I don't know…my life…what am I doing?"

"Samone are you worried about me telling Brian things about you both?" I didn't say anything.

"Well, if you are don't worry. He has tried to get some information out of me when he found out that you were my sister. I didn't tell him anything, but he surprised me when he told me that your name sounded familiar." I took my face out of my hands and looked at her.

"At first, he wouldn't tell me how your name sounded familiar to him, but I kept pressuring him to tell me. He told me that your name has come up in his investigation dealing with Joshua."

She grabbed my hand and said, "Sis let Charles take you away from here. Things are about to go down and I don't want you to be in the middle of it. Sometimes I think Brian is out to get you as well. He has said that you are an important factor to his case. I don't think he wants to take you to jail. I just think he wants to use you as his pawn to get close to Joshua."

I shook my head out of disbelief. Now I was truly frightened. Michelle was out to kill me; Brian was out to use me and Charles wanted to take me away somewhere that no one knew. If I ran away it wouldn't do any good because Brian was bound to find me.

"Get out of here Samone. Go with Charles, I'm sure he can keep you safe."

"I know that sounds like the best thing to do, but you just told me that Brian wants to use me as his pawn. Now you know he is going to follow me wherever I go."

She looked down at the floor and said, "You know what, you are right. He probably would follow you." Just then my phone rang.

It was 12:30 in the morning and no other was calling but Joshua Franks. Dedra looked at the phone then at me.

"Who is that?"

"Joshua," I exhaled and said, "let me answer this."

"You really shouldn't," my sister said.

I answered the phone with a dry hello.

"What's wrong Samone? I can hear it in your voice. Are you over your sister's house?"

"Yes, and I'm not doing so hot. I got mad stress in my life…"

Just then I remembered I didn't take my medicine. So I got up and grabbed my bag.

"…hold on Joshua."

I pulled out my medicine and headed toward the kitchen. I put one pill in my mouth and drowned it with water. I returned to cap to its rightful place.

"Hello…yeah I'm back." I looked for my sister who had gone to the back to her bedroom.

"Tell me Baby what's going on."

"Are you done with what you had to do?"

"Yeah, I'm at home right now."

"How long has it been since you have been done?"

"Well, I just made it home about 15 minutes ago. Now, how much longer are you going to keep me in suspense about you?"

"Well, it's this whole situation about Michelle. I don't know what to do about her."

"You don't have to do nothing but one thing." I was confused now because I didn't know what he was talking about.

"What's that?"

"All you got to do is say that you saw her kill this man named Lester Green."

"Who is Lester Green?"

"If I told you, you wouldn't agree to do it. Let's just say you are doing me a favor as well as getting Michelle off you back." I sat there and just stared at the wall. I almost forgot that I was on the phone.

"Hello. Samone are you there?"

"Oh, yeah. I'm here. And you got some damn nerves asking me to do something like that. I can't believe you would even consider me doing something like that without letting me know what for. Joshua what did you do?"

"What do you mean what did I do? I didn't do anything. And besides that you know I can't be talking personal business over the phone. You know what…I'm on my way over there."

"What do you mean? You make it seem as if you couldn't come over here. Tell me Baby what is going on? My life is at hand with this ordeal."

"I know what your life is…and I understand that you are afraid right now. I'm on my way. Just hold on Baby, I will be right there."

I wanted to see Joshua face to face to have a very detail conversation with him about this whole situation, but something in me told me to tell him not to come over. So I did.

"Joshua I don't think it's a great idea for you to come over here right now or ever for that reason."

"Why not, he asked?

"Because my sister is dating the assistant district attorney and he is very likely to just pop up over here."

"You mean Brian Johnson?"

"Don't pretend now…you know she is dating him. She told you before me."

I heard him mumble to himself…"I can't believe this shit."

"Um look, see if you can get your sister's car so you can meet me somewhere."

"Okay, I will see what I can do. I will call you back in like 15 minutes."

"A'ight, bet."

I pressed the end button on my cell phone and put the phone in my pocket. I slowly got up from the couch and exhaled. Hopefully, my sister wouldn't mind me using her car. I really needed to see Joshua to see what the hell was going on.

"Sista, I said through the door." I then knocked three times on the door.

"What do you want Samone? What, you want to use my car?" Believe it or not but somehow I was already expecting her to know what I wanted.

"Can I open the door?"

"Sure, why not?" my sister said out of disgust.

"Why do you sound so vexed with me?"

"Because Samone…you are still having dealings with that man. You know all he is trouble for you! Why can't you see that?" I walked over to the bed where my sister was under the covers lying down.

"Look, I know he is nothing but trouble, but he is my trouble."

Dedra interrupted me, "your trouble…that doesn't even make sense."

"What I meant, is that he may not be the most decent man in the world but he has been there for me. He was there for me when I needed him most. Yes, he is in trouble right now, but now my life is in trouble right along with his. I have to straighten this mess out before I'm ruined. Can't you understand that no one knows Joshua better than I do? I can get him to turn all this crap around."

She looked at me in the strangest way. She looked at me as if I were a ghost. That let me know that she didn't hear a word I just said.

"Okay, whatever you say Samone. I give up. Take the keys they are on the dresser beside my purse."

I was a little reluctant to get the keys off her dresser. She made me feel so idiotic because if the decision I made.

"I love you Dedra and don't ever forget that."

Dedra stared off into space and said, "How could I, you are my big sister and I love you too."

I knew she was about to start crying by the edge in her voice. I really didn't want to see my baby Sis start to cry so I exited the door with speed.

"Be careful Samone. I want to see you again!" I heard her yell behind me.

"I will," I yelled back.

Once outside, the chilly air brushed up against my face. The car was a little warmer inside than out. Once I turned the ignition on I felt something vibrate in my pocket.

"Hello."

"I thought you were going to call me back. Were you able to get the car?"

"Sorry Babe, my sister was on my mind. So where do you want to meet?"

"How about that basketball court around the corner of your sister's? I will be there in about 5 minutes. I took the liberty of leaving the house when we hung up the phone. I knew I had to see you tonight My Love."

"Okay, that's fine. I will be there in about 7 minutes."

I ended up making it in seven minutes exactly and Joshua's Lexus was already there. He jumped out of his car and ran to my sister's, which made me look around for I thought something was going on. Joshua opened the driver's door and pulled me out of the car.

"Joshua what is going on?" I looked at his face and he didn't look like anything was wrong. He took me in his arms and kissed me.

"Damn I'm so happy to see you. I missed you so much."

"Joshua don't do that shit to me. I thought something was going on the way you ran up to me like that." I pushed myself away from him and looked into his eyes.

"Now tell me about this Lester Green character."

"I will, but were you followed?"

"How should I know for sure? I'm not an investigator. From what I can tell, I wasn't."

"Okay, good then. Now when I tell you this you make sure you don't tell anyone else. I trust you Samone and you are the only someone I have right now. Tyrone is tripping and I know he wants my spot now."

My mouth opened and I was somehow surprised when I shouldn't have been. I mean, I knew what Tyrone was up to from the beginning.

"How do you know that?" I asked.

"Well, let me tell you about Lester Green first. Lester Green is the kingpin from the North side of town. He knew of me because..." He stopped at that and turned away.

"Don't stop now. Continue Joshua."

Joshua took a couple of steps away from me then said, "I can't believe I'm telling you all of this stuff. You are too innocent for the crime life. You may not need to know this stuff for your own good. This I have to tell you can hunt you for the rest of your life." I began to have mixed emotions, for I didn't know how to feel to that response.

"Joshua, what are you talking about?" Tears were in his eyes and he began to say something, but I couldn't hear him.

"...Lester Green is dead because of me," he hung his head low and sighed, "there I said it," he confessed. This eerie senseless feeling came over me. I sat down on my sister's car with the breath out of me.

"You what? Tell me it isn't so." Joshua walked to where I was and tried to console me.

"Get your hands off of me." I pushed him away from me.

I was in disbelief that he took a man's life. Now I know that is what gangstas do, but to hear him actually confess to a murder made me feel really uneasy.

"So you are going to leave me too? I told you in trust that you would understand why I need you. I love you. Please don't do me like this."

"Joshua, you killed a man. And now you want me to lie and say I saw someone else do it." Joshua now erased the tears from his eyes and became manlier.

"Samone, I had to. He was going to kill me if I didn't. Don't you know this dope game is for grabs? Everyone is out to get the money that is out there. Everyone is looking to take over different hoods and cities if they can. The more you lead the more money you make. Lester knew this and I know it."

"Tell me this, when did this happen and was Tyrone there with you?"

"This happened about six months ago. And yes, Tyrone was there with me. The case is just now being brought up because Johnson thinks he can get someone to say that they saw me. No one is confessing that they saw me because they are scared something may happen to them, but I'm afraid someone may break. I wouldn't ask you to do what I asked you to do if I felt different."

"Well, did someone see you or not?"

"To be honest the old lady may have seen me."

"How did you kill him?" Joshua looked at me with helplessness in the eyes.

"Does it really matter Samone?" I knew he really didn't want to talk about it anymore, so I left it at that.

"Nah, it doesn't matter at all." Joshua walked to my sister's car and placed his hands upon my waist.

"Hear me good Samone. And hear me with your heart. I'm sorry I got you mixed up in this mess. You always told me that something like this could happen and now it has. I just didn't know it would be like my own so called homie doing this to me," he exhaled and let the pressures of his mind slip through his mouth, "don't believe what others say about me, because you know me Samone, better than anyone. My life is going to change after this…" He let his hands drop to his waist and turned his face to face his car. "…if I make it out of this." I turned his face to face mine so that I could look into his eyes.

"What do you mean if you make it out of this? Look, we are both going to make it out of this alive and well. We have to believe and be smart about this situation."

Before I could finish my thoughts he said, "Samone I need you to witness to seeing Michelle doing the murder. I mean, that would get her off your back and she would be behind bars like she should be. Tyrone has told me of their ventures together doing devious things. I can't get all into their business right now for this is not the time, but I need this Baby please say that you will do it." I didn't know what to think. He was asking me to commit perjury.

"You do realize if I get caught committing perjury that I will go to jail? Brian will know the truth and spot it out and I will be stuck like chuck. I don't know Joshua…it's like you are asking me to do something without caring about the consequences. All you are doing is thinking about yourself. How selfish can you be?"

I expected Joshua to get angry and retaliate with words of frustration and pain, but he didn't. He just put his head in his hands.

With his hands to his side he said, "Alright, if that's your decision I have to live with it. You were my last hope of getting out of this situation. If I go to jail, it will be your fault."

"Oh hell no, you are not about to blame your mistakes and misfortunes on me. You made the decision to kill someone. Right now I am thinking of the trouble that I could get into with my actions. I thought you loved me. If you really loved me you wouldn't have ever put me in the position that you have now. I can't believe you. You got some nerves." With that I walked to the driver's side of my sister's car and opened the door.

Before I could get in Joshua grabbed my arm and slung me around to face him.

"Look here woman…I don't want you to ever think I never loved you. If I didn't love you I wouldn't have told you all the things that I have told you. I trusted you and I thought you loved me and would do anything for me."

"Joshua get your hands off of me…you are hurting my arm." He let go of my arm and I looked at it and found his handprint still in my arm.

"Now you look here…back in the day I probably would have done what you are asking me to do right now but I'm not that little ole girl anymore.

I'm a grown woman now and I'm making grown woman decisions for my life. I love you Joshua I really do and I really hope nothing happen to you, but I can't lie. I never was a good liar and you know that." He began to back up to his car.

Still looking at me he said, "I will never let anything happen to you Samone…I will still be there for you even though you refuse to do what I asked you to do."

"And I will be there for you in other ways…I'm sorry, I just can't do what you asked me to do."

Joshua got in his car and drove off like he had a serious attitude. Jumping back into my sister's car I began to think about how selfish he really was. I couldn't believe he thought I would risk putting my life in jeopardy for his. I was angry, hurt, confused, and lost in my thoughts that I didn't notice that another car had pulled up. The lights blinded me and I could not see who was in the other car. The greatest fear climbed in my skin and made goose bumps appear. With a nervous hand I started up the engine and put the car in reverse. I heard a male voice call out my name.

"Samone! Samone!"

I got so afraid that I slung that car around and drove away. I looked in the rearview mirror to see if the car followed me. The male must have gone his way because the streets seemed to be empty except for a couple of cars. My phone began to vibrate while I was doing seventy five on the express way.

"Hello." No answer.

"Hello. Who is this?" There was still no answer. I could tell that there was someone on the other end for I heard them breathing.

"Look, whoever this is stop calling my phone. Don't let me find out who this is for I will get the police involved."

After all my threats and persuasive words there was still no answer. So I hung up the phone. I began to think to myself who that may have been. It's so many people now that want a piece of me. And I don't entirely mean in a good way either.

Things could not get any worst, for when I made it back to my sister's Brian was there. As I entered the door I looked at my watch and it was after 2 a.m. It was late and I began to wonder why Brian was sitting on the couch with his legs crossed listening to my sister cry out.

"Ah ha…there she is…the lovely Samone Grey," Brain said with sarcasm.

"Brian, what a pleasant surprise to see you here at my sister's." Dedra got up from her seat. As she began to hug me she sighed with relief.

"I thought something had happened to you. Where have you been?"

While proceeding to stand up Brian opened his mouth again and said, "Dedra…Dedra just calm down. I'm quite sure that Samone here, has a perfect reason why she didn't call you and let you know that she was fine."

"Brian, let me handle this. She is my sister and I will be the one who will interrogate her." She turned her worried eyes back to face me.

"So, where were you?"

For some reason Brain's eyes became more intrigued than usual. I knew that I couldn't trust him. He was plotting out how to get me and Joshua. I mean, he really didn't have anything illegal on me, but he somehow knew that I knew all the dirt on Joshua. He was just itching to get that information. I walked between the two of them and sat down on the couch.

"Why do you want to know where I was? I'm here now and that is what matters."

I gave her the 'you better shut up look' so she could sit down. I guess she didn't catch on because she continued to question me.

"Samone, I need for you to tell me where you were tonight."

"Why Dedra why? What good is it going to be for you to know where I was tonight? I mean, why do you want to know so bad?"

I looked at Brian who began to exhale out of frustration. Then I knew what was going on. He wanted to know where I was tonight. Then it dawned on me. Could it have been Brian that was at the court after Joshua left? I didn't know but I was for sure going to find out.

"Wait a minute. When and why did you come here Brian?"

"Huh?"

"Huh is not the answer I was looking for. I asked you when and why did you come here?"

"I don't understand why you would want to know that. I'm here for your sister's sake. She called me with tears in her voice and I rushed over here to comfort her. Now it seems to me that you are avoiding the question that is asked of you."

"First of all, no one in this room is my mother or father so therefore my safety is in my own hands. Secondly, I don't need someone who I don't even know to try and get my sister to get information out of me. If you want to know something just ask me. Brian."

"See, I was trying to be nice and pleasant but you are about to see the gruesome side of me. I didn't want to show this side of me because of your sister, but I see now I have to show it."

"Show me what you will. Because I have a side to me as well."

"Oh, I bet you do. I mean, you wouldn't be dating that thug for no reason. I'm sure you do what you do when you are with him."

Before I knew it I was standing right in Brian's face and he was in my face. It was as if we were about to throw down.

"Why are you two so eager to fight? I know the both of you have an agenda as to doing what is right, but you don't have to go down this route. All that I ask is that you two somehow work together."

At that note, both Brian and I looked at my sister. I had an expression letting her know that that was out of the question and he had a look that described him as being ok with the idea.

"This situation has gotten out of control. I apologize baby for my behavior. I won't let it happen again."

"Sure you won't," I said. He grimaced and went to console Dedra.

"Let's get this straight Brian. I am Joshua's love and I don't see myself telling you information about him. So, if that was your plan, I'm sorry to disturb it, but that's just the way it is."

"Do you actually believe I was planning on getting information from you about Franks? That's not my plan at all. I have a totally different mentality than you. And I'm not about to sneak down to your level and perform the actions you think I qualify for."

"Ooo Wee Mr. Attorney At Law. Well, don't you have words. But for your information, in some way you are trying to get information from me. It may not be from me myself and I…" I turned and looked at my sister, "…but I have a hint as to whom you are trying to pursue getting information from." Brian licked his lips.

"I see you think you know what you are talking about, but this is my love right here. And I'm not trying to put her in any situation that may jeopardize our relationship. Talk to your boyfriend and maybe he will do the same for you." He hit me deep with that dagger. I couldn't say anything else. I left it at that.

"Whatever Brian." He kissed my sister on the forehead grabbed his hat and jacket then left.

"Man...he really stuck it to you with that one, huh?"

"Dedra the truth of the matter is that Brian put on a front. He knows what he is doing. He knows that he is getting his sources from you. That's why you wanted to know where I was tonight." Dedra turned from me and began to walk down the hallway to her bedroom.

"You may be right Samone...you may be right."

With that I went to the hall closet and got my blanket and pillow, laid on the couch and went to sleep. Tomorrow or better yet today is my last day off before I go back to work. With all the drama and misfortunes going on, I really don't know how I will respond to working. We will see though. Hopefully, life gets better than this.

Love's Mirage

CHAPTER SIX

The next morning, I found a letter from my sister on the table beside me. It read, *Hey Sis, by the time you get this I will be gone to work. I hope you understand that I had to go. I don't have no one else to pay my bills yet like you do. Anyhow, just call me on my cell if you need anything. There is a key on the kitchen counter if you wish to leave the house, please lock up. P.S. try to contact Charles maybe he can get you out of here. Love Ya, Sis.*

I folded the letter back up and place it back on the table. I look around the environment that I was shortly relocated to. It was very peaceful and homey. My sister had pretty good taste as well. Her living room set consisted of red, black, and white plaid furniture, three piece gold trimmed glass tables, and pictures galore. My sister must have a fetish with pictures because they were all on her walls and on her tables. There were pictures of our family, her friends, and she even had a picture of Brian. I'm not really that big on pictures, but I do have a few up in my apartment. I looked at her center table and realized a center piece that involved pictures. The rainbow glass object had departments where pictures went. It spelled out my sister's name. She must have had this thing custom built because I didn't see anything like this in stores. I tried to pick it up but it was heavy, so I placed it back down in its rightful place. I counted the departments on each letter to get a total count of pictures. There was 37 places to put pictures and every one of them had a picture.

"Hmm, very creative." Whoever thought of this did a good job.

My eyes wondered the room then landed on the television. I found the remote on the couch and flicked it on. The first thing that I heard advertised was diet pills. The world must really be out of shape because that's all you see on television these days. I flicked to the next channel and the news was on. I turned the volume up and waited to see what the topic was about.

"Hello, Austin. This is Bradley Moore with the criminal case of Joshua Franks…" Oh my God. I couldn't believe that Joshua was on T.V. Why didn't he tell me that his case would be exposed to millions.

"…apparently the jury cannot make a unanimous decision on if Joshua Franks should be put in jail. Assistant District Attorney Brian Johnson has delivered powerful evidence against Joshua Franks and has concluded that Joshua Franks should be put behind bars."

I watched on as they showed Brian introduce evidence to the case. I must admit he is a very attractive man. I don't know how old he is but he looked to be in his thirties. The witness that Brian was interrogating was a white woman who happened to be a senior citizen. Brian drilled her hard with questions about the evidence of bullet shells that were left at the scene.

"Now, Mrs. Boston. These are the bullet shells that were found at the scene of the murder. You do remember seeing the murderer holding a gun, right?"

Just as the witness was about to answer, Bradley Moore came back onto the screen saying that he wasn't sure how long the case would be in court. "…I will keep you posted on the progress of this case. This is Bradley Moore with channel seven news."

I will never forget the image of Joshua sitting there with his chin between his fingers. He tried to play everything off by staying in a state of tranquility. Joshua was dressed in a light blue suit with a yellow and blue tie that matched. It fit him very well. Actually, I remember that suit from an event that we attended the year before. He still looks nice in it like the first day that he wore it.

I sat down on the couch to sort out my thoughts about Joshua's case being on the news.

"I knew it."

For some strange reason I knew that Brian was on the case. I wasn't surprised to see him at all. So far it looks like the case may end up being a mistrial. There are no real witnesses and evidence that pin-point Joshua to the murder. I can see why the jury may have a hard time coming up with an agreement. Hopefully, they don't just judge him because of his background. Many people do. To tell you the truth, I even judge him. Joshua is really nothing but trouble for me, but I continue to try and love him in hopes that we will one day be a happy couple. I don't know if that will ever happen but hopefully it will. I'm not giving up on Joshua yet. Somehow though, I am going to have to figure out a way to keep Charles. However, I know Charles is not the one to string along. I need to figure out which one I want to be with and I need to figure this out fast. I don't know how much longer my emotions can stand to be split. I realized that I was wasting time sitting on the couch and looking around, so I got up and walked to the bathroom. Seeing my reflection made me give out a groan. I looked horrible. I guess I had a bad reaction to the medication or something because my eyes were the color of scarlet and they also had big bags under them. I rinsed my eyes out with water, hoping that would help. Luckily, they didn't burn. I pulled my hair back into a ponytail, which made me look younger, then I proceeding on putting make-up on. It was a good thing that my sister and I enjoy the same color of make-up, because I would have been in a world of trouble. The make-up really helped my eyes, it covered the bags and the water made the puffiness go away. It took me 30 minutes in all to get dressed, which I think is pretty good, a lot of women take longer than that to get dressed. After primping in the mirror for 30 minutes I got hungry. The kitchen was big enough to fit three people at a time in it which was impressive for an apartment. I opened the refrigerator and pulled out the eggs, turkey bacon, and cheese. After I ate my quick fix of a breakfast, my sister's home phone rang. The answering machine picked up and I heard Dedra's voice through the speakers saying...*Sorry I'm not home right now but do leave your name and a brief message and I will return your call as soon as possible thank you.*

"Hello, Ms. Grey. This is Captain Haynes with the Austin Police Department. We have news that a Samone Grey is staying with you right now. Please inform her that we are looking to speak with her about an investigation. Thank you." I froze.

The glass of orange juice in my hand began to shake with my hand. The first thing that I could think of was to call Charles. But I didn't instead I called Joshua. He answered the phone with three rings.

"Joshua. Why in the hell is the cops looking for me?"

"What!?! Samone what are you talking about?"

"Joshua I swear, I was just finishing my glass of orange juice and the Captain of the Austin Police Department left a message to my sister to inform me that they wish to speak with me."

"I don't know why they are looking for you." The weirdest feeling came over me. I felt that Joshua was telling me a lie.

"Come on now Joshua, if you know something you better tell me."

"I swear to you that I don't know anything. If it makes you feel any better they are looking to speak with me again. I know you must have seen my case on the news by now. I have to meet in court again today at three. I would like for you to be there if you can."

"Joshua, I just told you that the police are looking for me and you are talking about yourself. It's like you don't care anymore. You are changing into this man that I don't know." There was silence over the phone and the next thing I know, I got the dial tone.

"Hello. Hello. Joshua, are you there." It didn't make any sense for me to continue to talk to the dial tone, so I hung up.

That's strange; that has never happened with Joshua talking to me. I figured it was a dropped call, so I call his number again. This time a woman answered the phone.

"Hello. Who is this?"

"Is Joshua there?"

"Yes, he is here, but what I would like to know is, who are you? Is this the bitch he claims he in love with?"

"Hold on, wait a minute. I'm no bitch and I don't appreciate you calling me one…"

I was flabbergasted to the fact that another woman was answering my man's phone and insulting me. I couldn't believe that this was happening. "…now put Joshua on the phone."

I don't know if it was my tone or if it was just Joshua snatching the phone, but he answered the phone with, "Baby, I'm sorry."

"You are sorry Joshua. You are one sorry man. Here I am, being faithful to you and you cheating on me with some woman. I can't believe you. I knew you were doing something. I just knew it. Look, you don't have to worry about me. I see you found someone else."

"Nah, Baby it's not..." Before he finished, I snap my phone back in its rightful position.

The jingle on my phone kept playing for about 5 minutes. He must have called me at least 10 times straight. I wasn't having that. I wasn't about to give in and answer his call so he could just lie to me. It felt like the world was crashing down on me. All this bad stuff was happening to me all at once. I began to pace the room and tried to sort things out. I tried to put things together like that of a jigsaw puzzle when I suddenly saw a letter on the floor by the front door. Someone had slid the note under the door.

I exhaled, I looked up to the ceiling to face Heaven and said, "Lord, what more can happen?"

I picked up the letter and it had my name on it in big letters. I opened it and it read,

I've been waiting on your call, but you never called me. I would appreciate it if you would call me instead of your man. Here is the number again 512-555-9560, call me asap. I sat down on the couch and began to cry.

What in the world did this creep want? I had the letter in one hand and the phone in the other, but I thought to myself, *"should I call this number?"*

I re-read the letter again and realized that the only person that could have known the number to call was Charles. Joshua didn't know anything about the other letter. I dialed Charles's cell phone number.

"Bout time you call. What took you so long?"

"Charles, I really don't need to hear that right now. All I need for you to do is answer my question."

"And what is dat?"

"Did you keep that letter that day with the number on it and if you did, did you call it?"

"What letta?"

"Don't play Charles. You know what letter I'm talking about."

"Oh dat' letta. Yeah, wha's it to you?"

"Don't worry about all that. Just answer this last question. Who was it and what did they want?"

"Samone, that's two questions." He let out a little laugh.

"Look, Charles I don't got time for games. Tell me what I want to know."

"A'ight. Man, I was just kiddin' around. Well, wen' I called the numba. Some woman answered da phone. She said she needed to speak with chu' and only you. She wouldn't giv' me any info about nuthin'."

I began to ponder on what Charles just told me. It didn't make sense. The Austin Police Department, Tyrone, Michelle, Brian, Charles, and now this mystery woman wanted a piece of me. Why me? What did I do that was so bad?

"Samone, I really think chu should call her. Just get it out of the way. Find out wha she want."

"You right, Charles I am going to call her. And by the way, what else have you found out about me Charles? You seem to know me better than I know myself these days."

"Well, I'm not gon' say I know everything bout you, but I know most of what is going on. You need to watch out for that no good boyfriend of yours."

I thought about telling Charles that Joshua and I are no longer together, but I decided differently. He may get too excited about the whole ordeal.

"Well, Charles that is the reason I called you. I think I'm about to call this mystery woman now. So I will chat with you later."

"Before you go…are you gonna' go away with me or what? I need to know."

"I will let you know. I may have to take you up on your offer."

"Wow! I can't believe you are talking with some sense now. I was expecting you to say no."

"Well, I have so much going on in my life that I just may have to run away to just clear my head."

"I'm here for you Baby…just know that I am. Okay?"

"Okay. Bye Charles."

"Bye Baby."

After talking with Charles and hearing him reassure me that he was there for me, it made me feel so much better. Charles is a good man. I mean, he would be there for me if only I let him. With Joshua having another woman I should take Charles in my arms and allow us to be in love. But hey, I don't know. If I decide to be with Charles things may not be what I expect. So, for now I'm going to be by myself and try and get all this drama out of my life on my own. I don't know how I'm going to do it, but I am. First thing first, I need to find out who this woman is and what she wanted with me, then I'm going to call that Captain Haynes character. I began to push the buttons on my phone and there was a ring. A woman answered the phone with the sweetest voice. It was one of those voices that you could just listen to for hours.

"Hello."

"Yeah, this is Samone. I got your letter and I just wanted to know what this is all about."

"Oh, so you finally called. I'm glad. There is so much to tell you, but I would prefer to talk in person."

"Well, I would like to know who this is, how you found me, and why do we have to meet? I mean, you can just tell me what you need to tell me over the phone. You got to understand that I don't know you and you seem to know who I am and it's pretty spooky."

"Okay. I give you that and I understand where you are coming from. So, I will just break down what I know to you over the phone."

"Well, thank you. So, who are you?"

"My name is Janice Carlbright with The Channel 7 News. I have been trying to contact you for a while now. As you may know, I have a sister by the name of Michelle Carlbright. I'm sorry to break this news to you but she is planning to kill you. I'm working with the Austin Police Department about this situation. You may have received a phone call by someone name Captain Haynes. My sister has no clue as to what I'm doing. If she did she would probably harm me as well."

"Wait, wait wait….hold on. You mean to tell me you would risk your life to save mine and you don't even know me? Why?"

"Yes. I feel you didn't do anything to deserve death, so I planned to intervene. Michelle and her fiancé Tyrone have been planning to kill you and Joshua for at least three months now. I overheard her on a couple of occasions, talking to Tyrone. I even recorded a couple of their conversations. The only problem with the recorded conversations is that they never mention any names. They talk in code and it has left the police department with very few options on making an arrest. Sad to say, my sister Michelle has a split personality. One minute she is sweet as honey, then the next she hates the world. Lately, though, she has been the aggressive type. She hates the world and everyone in it except Tyrone. She loves what he is about because he is the same way. I don't know if he suffers from having a split personality, but I do know that he wants to see both of you dead." I was pacing the floor while Janice spilled the goods to me. All the while, I was trying to put the pieces together.

"Michelle never told me that she suffers from having a split personality."

"She wouldn't; she is in denial about the whole diagnosis."

Knowing that bit of information explains everything. It explained how she used to seem different at times. I couldn't put my finger on it, but I always knew there was something about her that wasn't right.

"Is she on any medication?"

"Well, she is supposed to be, but she doesn't take it regularly. She takes it when she wants to. But now I don't think she takes it at all."

"So, what did you tell Captain Haynes?"

"Oh, I told him that your life is in danger and that you need surveillance."

"How did you find me now?"

"I'm a journalist. I have my ways of getting information. You talk to the right people; you are bound to get the information that you desire."

"Did Captain Haynes go for the news you told him?"

"Of course he did, me and him go way back. He is a dear friend to me."

"Well, Janice I do thank you for your helping me and looking out for me. I will repay you somehow."

"Don't worry about repaying me. This is for free. I remember how my sister used to speak of you at dinner. She used to say such nice things. Now she doesn't say a word. She doesn't even show up half the time. When she does show up she is hostile and violent. My father and mother don't want to have anything to do with her; until she starts taking her medicine. The only time she gets aggressive is when she doesn't take her medicine. So, everyone in the family knows what is going on. I hope this bit of information helps you and if you need me just call."

"I will and thank you so much for the warning."

"You are welcome. Be sure to call Captain Haynes… okay?"

"Okay, I'm about to call him right now." We both hung up.

It's amazing how God works. I was just stressing about how I was going to clear my life of drama and here Janice was already working on my behalf. My phone rang…

"Hello. What do you want Joshua? I have nothing to say to you."

"It's not what you have to say to me…it's what I have to say to you. First, let me say this…that woman that answered the phone was someone from my past. Yes, I did sleep with her, but it was at the beginning of our relationship. She is trying to get back in my life, but I continue to tell her that I'm in love with you. She knows about you. I'm not telling no lie when I say this either, there is NOTHING going on between us."

"If that is so true Joshua…why is she still calling you and why is she going to your house answering your damn phone? Why is she still in your life period?" There was silence over the phone and it made me suspect that he was lying.

"See Joshua, I knew your ass was lying…don't ever call me again."

He then answered me with this pathetic energy, "It's not a lie…and the reason why she still in my life is because there is a kid involved."

"What!?! What do you mean there is a kid involved? You mean to tell me that you are a father? When were you going to tell me, huh? When Joshua?"

"I couldn't find the best time to tell you. I was going to tell you at Chili's when we had dinner, but other stuff came up. I'm truly sorry Samone."

"Tell me, is the kid yours?"

"I don't know. I'm going to get a DNA test done next week when I'm done with all my court dates. Look, Samone I never meant to hurt you, but this shit just happened. I didn't plan for all of this to happen."

"So, why did you cheat on me? Wasn't I good enough?"

"You are perfect for me…it's just…well…I was drunk. I remember throwing a party for Lance and she was there. She kept pestering me. I mean, she stayed in my face the whole night and when I finally got drunk, it happened."

"So, your ass didn't use protection?"

"Yeah, I did."

"Don't lie Joshua. Did you?"

"Honestly, Samone I don't remember. I do remember asking her if she had one."

"Oooo…," I said with frustration, "…who knows what that hoe got Joshua….I can't believe you." He didn't say anything else; he just sat there and took all that I had to say.

"Look, I will call you when I feel like it. Until then, you get your shit together. Bye Joshua." With that, I closed the flip phone.

Joshua could really be a father now. According to Joshua's slip up the child should be at least one and a half to two-years-old. I know that whore told Joshua she was pregnant when she first found out. He chose to keep this shit a secret for this long. I couldn't believe his ass. If it's not one thing, it's another. I didn't get to tell him the information that I had recently found out from Janice. I no longer wanted to be on the phone with him. I was having all kinds of thoughts running through my brain. They kept coming one after another. I thought I was having a nervous breakdown.

As I began to think about Joshua's issue again, the puzzle began to look finished to me. I mean, it explained why he has been so distant lately. I've wanted him to stay the night with me lately and he has been turning me down. I guess that whore has really been in his face again. I mean, this is all of a sudden. Maybe he stopped given her the money that she desired.

I wanted to ask him a lot of questions, but I refuse to call him back. My pride wouldn't let me do such a thing. I just sat there and looked at the television. As usual there was a diet commercial playing. I changed the channel and the Steve Wilkos show was on. There were 30 minutes left to the show and apparently, the show was about a father being accused of molesting his daughter.

"It's so sad what people go through in life," I thought to myself.

"I think you did it…just admit it. You molested your child. You pervert. You freak." Steve was in the man's face and he was calling him all kinds of names.

The man just retorted, "I'm not a child molester and I didn't do it."

"We will see what the lie detector test shows. How about that?" Steve said.

I thought to myself, *"One day Steve is going to get hit. He is always in someone's face."*

"You know what…why don't you molest me? Do it to me. No…you are afraid to pick on someone your own size."

The man just stood there and took all the insults; he didn't say a word. I guess he figured he said all he could say to try and convince Steve and the audience. As I was watching the television, my phone rang again. The caller ID announced that it was my supervisor, Brenda Jackson. Both my eyebrows rose with astonishment. I wonder what she wanted.

"Hello."

"Hi Samone."

"Hi Brenda."

"Well, I know you are wondering why I am calling you. The reason is I received a phone call from a young lady and she told me some surprising news about you. I called you to find out for myself if the news was true."

"Brenda, I hate to interrupt you but did you get the name of the young lady?"

"No. She said she would rather leave herself to be anonymous."

"Oh."

"Well, as I was saying…she told me some things about you that I found to be alarming."

"Oh really? Well, what did she tell you?"

"She told me that you were into drugs and that you had a mental disorder because of the drugs. Is this true?" When she told me that I knew exactly who told her the lies.

"Brenda, I just want you to know that none of what she told you are true except for one thing. I have been diagnosed with schizoaffective disorder."

"Oh my. What is that Samone?"

"It's when a person is in between being schizophrenic and having bipolar disorder. I'm currently on medication right now that helps me with the symptoms. I also want you to know that this will not affect my job performance. I have a lot going on in my life right now and I'm just trying to cope with life." Brenda was quiet for a while. I guess she was deciding on whether or not if she wanted me to return to work.

"Samone, are you sure you are not taking any drugs?"

"What? Drugs? Oh no, you have me greatly misunderstood. I don't take any drugs except the ones that are prescribed to me. You have to believe me."

"Well, I just want you to know that the young lady was very convincing in what she was saying about you. She said that you would tell me that you were fine and that you don't do drugs. She also said that I shouldn't believe a word you said. I have my own image of you Samone and it doesn't involve drugs. I was worried about you when you called me that day. I knew something was totally wrong. I felt it within my spirit. Look, I tell you what, how about you return to work when you get yourself together. No matter how long it takes you have your job waiting for you. You are an excellent worker and everyone gets along with you. Even the "bulldog" gets along with you..." She let out a little laugh at what she had just said. "...I know the nickname you all have given her, you may not know this, but she likes you. You are very well respected within the office. And I hope you have a speedy recovery. Take care Samone and I will talk with you later."

"Thank you so much Brenda. I really appreciate this."

"No problem."

I knew there was a reason why God sent me to that place of employment. Brenda really didn't have to do what she had just done. It's amazing how God works. Now I didn't have to worry about going to work. I had time to clear up these other mishaps.

It was two o' clock in the afternoon. It was the perfect time to all Captain Haynes. Hopefully, he will be able to help me out of this situation. I replayed the message off the answering machine. He didn't leave a number for me to return his call. Just as I was dialing the number to the Austin Police Department I heard someone on the receiver end saying hello.

"Hello," I officially answered the phone.

"Hey Sis, I was just calling to check up on you. I wanted to make sure that you were alright."

"Aww how sweet. I'm doing fine. I just got off the phone with my boss and she told me that I could return to work whenever I get myself together. And get this…she said it doesn't matter how long it takes and that my job will be there waiting for me. Isn't that great?"

"Yeah! That is really good news. Now you don't have to stress about going back so soon. Honestly, I think it's for the best. You got so much going on in your life right now."

"I know, isn't that the truth. I am so glad that you called Dedra; I needed to hear a friendly voice."

"I'm glad that you are okay right now. Did you remember to take your medicine last night?"

"Um, yes I did."

"Have you talked to that no good loser?"

"Yeah, I talked to him but I don't really want to talk about him right now. Guess who I did talk to though."

"Who? Charles?"

"Yeah, how did you know?"

"Well, don't get mad okay, he called me and told me that you called him. He was so excited."

"Why would I get mad at you because he called you? Now what you should have been saying is don't get jealous…because that I am right now."

"Why Sista?…don't be like that. All he thinks about is you." I let out a little laugh as to die down the uncomfortable vibe that was shifting from her to me and me to her.

"I'm only kidding with you Dedra. When did you become so serious?"

"Well, for a minute there it sounded like you were serious."

Little does she know I was serious. I must admit I'm jealous when it comes to Charles. Some time now I have noticed their little relationship blossom into something special. I could tell that she thought of it being a special relationship because every time we talk about him she gets this twinkle in her eye.

"Hello. See Samone you are serious. You are so quiet over the phone."

"Oh Girl stop. I was only thinking. You know I always think before I speak."

"Well, okay I was only checking. I don't want you to get upset with me about anything."

"I'm not angry, honestly, I'm okay."

"Good. Well, I am about to get back to work. I shall chat with you later."

"Okay. Bye."

"Bye."

I swear I better get with Charles before my sister does. It seems to me that's what she really wants. Are maybe I was just being paranoid. After talking with my sister I dialed the Austin Police Department to speak with Captain Haynes.

"Austin Police Department. How may I direct your call?"

"Captain Haynes, please."

"Sure thing."

I waited a couple of seconds and the phone began to ring. I was just about to hang up the phone when I heard a deep husky voice answer the phone.

"Captain Haynes speaking."

He spoke with a strong southern accent. In a way it reminded me of Charles. Or maybe Charles was just on my mind.

"Hello, how may I help you?"

"Oh, I'm sorry. My name is Samone Grey. My sister told me that you called her house today looking for me."

"Oh yes. Ms. Grey. It is alright for me to call you Ms. Grey, right?"

"Sure."

"Well, I'm just going to be blunt with the whole situation. It has been mentioned to me that someone is out to harm you. I was just calling you to make sure that these accusations were true."

"Well, Captain Haynes I'm sorry to say that they are correct."

"Okay. I have to ask you a few questions then. Let me grab a pen and paper."

I waited while he was rummaging. I knew he was about to ask me questions that I didn't and couldn't answer right now. I also knew the questions would lead up to Joshua because he was the key to everything. I debated on whether or not I was going to snitch on him. Nah, I couldn't go through with it. After all Joshua had done to me I was still thinking about his freedom and life.

"Um, excuse me, Captain Haynes, but I have to admit that there has been some misunderstanding. Some things aren't the way that they have been told to you. I'm sure that I will not need any help at this moment. Please forgive me for the confusion."

"What are you talking about, young lady? Are you sure you want to do this? I have good sources on this and to be frank I think you are just trying to cover for someone. Don't do it young lady. You have to remember your life and what it stands for. You have your whole life ahead of you and much is to be done with it, so take a few minutes and think about what you are doing right now." He was right to the point. He knew exactly what I was doing; I couldn't let him know that he was right though.

"I'm sure of what I'm doing Captain Haynes. I don't want to waste anymore of you time, please forgive me."

"Oh alright. I tried to warn you. You will probably need my help so keep my number handy. I usually leave the office late, so call me when you need me." With that, he hung up the phone.

I looked at the phones as if it were its fault for hanging up in my face.

"Samone get a grip on life." I said to myself.

I just turned down the best offer of help I have had since this mess began.

Now I was back to square one. It seemed as if I didn't want to live through this. I didn't know what kind of plan Michelle and Tyrone had come up with. They are murderers and I'm not. What defense do I have against them? I knew Janice was going to be disappointed at my decision not to take up Captain Haynes's offer of help. She put her life on the line just to get me that information and I just threw it all away. How was I going to get out of this without snitching on Joshua? A part of me wanted to just tell what I knew to the cops and the other wanted me to hold out to the end. Maybe I was still that young little girl who could not make good decisions. I'm so stuck on Joshua like glue but he doesn't realize it because he is so caught up with himself. I can't blame him because he does have a lot going on in his life, but damn so do I. The only two things that I got good going for me is the fact that I know Tyrone and Michelle are up to no good. The second thing is I could run away with Charles and probably live happily ever after. I sat down on the couch and began to contemplate on how I could get Michelle and Tyrone before they could get me. *"Maybe I could set Michelle up somehow,"* but how I wondered. Nothing was coming to me so I just sat there on that couch and watched TV. Clicking through the channels made me aware of how harmless I really was. I wasn't used to coming up with ways to disfigure someone's life and health. Let's just face it...I'm in trouble and I knew it.

Just as I was getting up to go to the bathroom; there was a knock on the door. The life almost went out of me, I was so shocked. Who would be at the door of my sister's place at this time of day? I knew it wasn't someone she knew because they knew she was at work. It never dawned on me till now that I could be putting my sister's life in jeopardy as well by living here. I knew I couldn't live here that much longer. I would have to go back to my place and face things out.

"Mmph, yeah right. I'm not going to be alone by myself waiting for death to stare me in the face." I pulled all the nerves I had in me together to answer the door.

"Who is it?" I said through the door.

"Ah-ha Ms. Grey, I see that you are still here. Please let me in."

"Um, you still didn't tell me who you were." Even though I already knew who it was, I wanted to give him a hard time.

"It's me Ms. Grey. Brian Johnson. Now could you please open the door so that we can chat."

"What do we need to chat about?"

"Open the door Ms. Grey." I slowly opened the door and he stepped in.

He had on a dark blue suit, white shirt, a tie with a silver horse and dark blue background, and dark blue shoes that matched the tie. I inhaled his scent and one of my eyebrows rose with satisfaction that he smelled really good. I looked at his hands and his nails were freshly manicured. Damn this man was fine. I didn't understand why he was here though. His woman wasn't here; what did he need to talk to me about? We already had the discussion of where he was going to get his information from about Joshua.

"I took a chance that you were still here Samone."

I let out a little yelp because of the way he said my name. That was the first time he really just said my name in a sentence, so it sounded really really nice.

"Is it just me or is it hot in here?" Brian let out a little laugh.

I didn't realize how close we were standing until he put my face within his hands and kissed me. I couldn't help it; I began to kiss back. His lips were so soft I thought I was kissing marshmallows.

I pushed him back after about two minutes of kissing and said, "Wait…wait a minute. What are we doing here?"

I heard him take in a deep breath and when he let the air go he said, "I've been wanting to do that since the very first time I laid my eyes on you."

"Brian. You know what we just did was wrong. But yet, I still want to do it again." This time one of his eyebrows rose; he scratched his head.

"Look Samone, I'm not here to lie to you. I find you extremely attractive and I'm not just talking about looks here. I'm talking about your character, your demeanor, and your willingness to be down for your man. I respect that about you." I didn't know what to say or think of that reason.

"Look, Brian you are my sister's man and that's that." Brian began to rub his chin as he thought about what I had just said.

"What if I told you that I love your sister but I didn't want her?"

"Honestly, I think you are infatuated with me for this short time but eventually you will want my sister back. Therefore, we don't need to do anything else."

"Well, since we are being honest here…when I first learned about you through my case, I thought of you as being a despicable person. I mean let's face it, you are dating someone who is very foul to our judicial system. He is one of the biggest drug lords in our city and believe it or not, he is a very dangerous man," Brian began to take steps to get closer to me, "he doesn't deserve someone like you." He reached for my face again but I moved.

"Look Brian, you can't be coming on to me like this." He placed a confused look on his face.

"Why not? Let me tell you something about me. When I see and want something I go after it until I get it. And maybe I want you right now."

"I don't know who you think you are but I am not the one. I have too much going on in my life right now and I don't need my sister's man trying to get at me. And to be honest I thought you hated me because I'm not giving you what you want."

"Samone I never hated you. I love that sassiness about you and that quick whipped mouthpiece of yours. Since you brought it up though, what is it that I want?"

"Brian. I don't know what this is, but you need to check yourself. You are wanting too much right now. You want me, my sister, and Joshua Franks behind bars. You need to play your hand right and do the right thing. Let's not hurt my sister. She is such a good person and she really loves you. I think you are just using me to get to Joshua anyway."

"So, do you actually think that I'm trying to come on to you to crack my case?"

I thought about what he asked me, "Um maybe. I don't really know that's what I'm trying to find out."

"Well, there is entirely nothing to consider. I told you the truth. Even though lawyers, prosecutors, and lawmakers are not considered honest people you have to believe me. And I'm not using you to get to Joshua. I'm the best at what I do and I don't need your help. I told you that we have different mentalities."

"So, what are you saying? I mean, what you are trying to do with me?"

"I'm saying that I love your sister for her honesty, sweetness, and loving kindness, but you…well let's just say I want you right now."

"Why? My sister has a much more stable life. She is also beautiful and most of all she cares for you."

I couldn't believe this. Charles, Joshua, and now Brian wanted little ole me. Well, I don't really know about Joshua anymore since he has that child now, but he swears that he is still in love with me. This is too much for one woman to take.

"Brian don't do this to me. Say it isn't so."

"I told you…I'm telling you the truth. It's hurting me to do this to your sister, but I can't get you out of my mind. I think about you late at night when there is no one around. I think about making love to you and spoiling you with my love. I understand what you are saying to me about Dedra. She is my world. Damn this is hard…" He sat down on the couch and exhaled a couple of times before he finished his sentence. "…I'm split between two sisters. I know which one I really want, but I don't want to hurt the other one."

"I hate to tell you this…I really do, but you want the wrong one. I'm not right for you. I have too much going on in my life. Settle down with someone who does not have the drama that I have."

He stood up and said, "I could care less about what is going on in your life. I could help you free yourself of those problems. Just say the word."

While I was exhaling large quantities of air I thought about the tears my sister would accumulate if she knew Brian's heart. To be truthful I desired him. A part of me just wanted to rip his clothes off and take him but I couldn't do it; I loved my sister too much. I haven't had a man of his stature ever approach me. It made me think what was it that made these men want me?

"I know how we can do this." Light of excitement grew in his eyes.

"You do? How?"

"We can never see each other again," I said turning my head.

His reaction was disappointment. He came close to where I was standing. I then took a seat on the loveseat. Like a lost puppy he followed; he sat down next to me.

"Samone that's not possible, I have to see you."

"No Brian. You have to see Dedra."

"So, it's like that?" Before I could answer the door swung open and my sister stepped through.

"Wow, what a wonderful surprise. Brian I wasn't expecting you to be here."

My sister ran over to Brian who was standing waiting for her hug. They hugged and kissed. Then Brian looked at me with pleading eyes. I couldn't figure out what he was pleading about. Maybe it was because he didn't want me to tell my sister what was said.

"So, Brian what are you doing here?"

"Oh, I was just in the neighborhood and I knew you were about to get off work so I stopped by." She looked at the both of us looking at one another.

"Is there something I should know," she asked.

We both replied, "No." at the same time.

She smiled and responded by saying, "I can't believe you two are getting along so well right now. Usually you two would be down each other's throats with smart remarks."

Before my sister could get any ideas about the two of us I said, "Oh, Brian and I have put our differences aside. We both knew it bothered you so we decided to stop quarreling so much."

"Oh really? This was done because of me?"

Then Brian added his two cents, "Yes, I want you to be happy and so does Samone."

Brian gave me an eye that let me know that he wasn't finish with what he started with me. I then gave him the eye that we were finished and I head motioned toward my sister to let him know why.

"What's up with you two? Y'all are both giving each other the eye and being so nice to one another. It makes me wonder if you two got something up." While my sister was still in Brian's left arm; he put his right arm around her then he whispered something in her ear.

It must have been something good because she giggled and said, "Okay, I will leave you two alone about this whole situation," she looked at me with her big smile, "well, I'm about to go and change really quickly. I will be done in a flash, so be ready when I come out Brian."

She left us alone which I really didn't want her to do. I knew Brian was going to say or do something I didn't want him to do.

"This is not over Samone. We still have to discuss this."

"Brian there is nothing to discuss. We did what we did and now it's over."

"Look, I know you want me. I can see it in your eyes. Stop playing or kidding yourself."

"Even if I did…"

"Okay, I'm ready," my sister said, stepping into the living room.

Brian put a smile on his face and replied, "My goodness that was fast."

"I know. My sister and I both share the same trait." Dedra laughed; then went to stand by Brian.

"You have made me so happy right now Brian. I can't believe you are actually taking me there " I was curious now.

She always wanted to go to some expensive restaurant on the North side of Austin, but no one she ever dated was able to afford it. She looked at me with exhilaration in her eyes.

"You know that new place I told you about Samone. Exquisite. Well, Brian has decided to take me there tonight."

"Oh really?" I asked.

"Yep. We will probably be late getting in tonight so don't wait up."

The whole time she was talking to me Brian was looking at me. He made sure he looked away when she looked at him though.

"Okay. Well, you two have fun."

I guess my situation crept up in her thoughts because she made a discomforting face, "Oh I almost forgot….will you be okay Samone?"

"Yeah, I will be fine Take care of my sister Brian."

"Oh she is in good hands."

Before they left Brian and I both acknowledged that my sister looked very pleasing to the eye. She had slipped on a short sleeved red dress that had a puffy bottom. The torso part of the dress was tight and had traces of lace in it. The red pumps that she had on matched perfectly. I don't see when she was able to put on some red eye shadow. I was even impressed with on how short it took her. After we said our compliments she blushed and thanked us both. Immediately afterwards, they left the apartment with high hopes of having a great experience at Exquisite. I watched through the window as Brian opened the passenger door for my sister. As he was walking to the other side of the car, I noticed him look back at the apartment. I wondered what he must have been thinking. Here my sister was happy as can be and he probably was thinking about me. He backed out of the parking space and zoomed off. I really did hope that they enjoyed themselves. They made a very attractive couple. It really didn't make sense to me about how we were at each other's throat, then turn around and kiss each other. I was so confused. I didn't know what life had next for me. But I knew I had to get away from my sister's place.

CHAPTER SEVEN

"Joshua please call me back. I need to talk to you." I ended the call and laid back on the couch.

I began to think about what could happen if Brain and I did start dating. I knew it would hurt my sister so very awful. Images of us escalate within my mind. Thoughts of us walking in the parks and having picnics. I tried to keep my thoughts clean but I couldn't help about thinking about the good love we would make when we did do something. His kiss told it all. I could tell that he knew what to do in the bedroom. I couldn't escape from his words that he spoke to me. They kept replaying in my head like a recorder. I looked at the ceiling and said a short prayer, Lord give me strength to endure all of the drama in my life. A sense of peace came over me and it felt good. It was the best feeling I had in a while.

"Thank you Lord for your peace."

I felt that I had a relationship with God even though I didn't attend church like I should. My mother was always on me about that. I prayed, read my Bible, and tried to be a good Christian. Nowadays though, it's pretty hard. The TV was still going while I closed my eyes. I began to become impatient about Joshua calling me back, so I dialed his number again.

Surprisingly, he answered, "What is it Samone?" I was startled by his pathetic composure that I asked with such demanding emotion.

"Why do you have to answer the phone like that? What did I do to you?"

"You should know what you did to me Samone. You left me hanging twice in a row."

"What?..." I almost yelled. "...how have I left you hanging twice?" I thought about it for myself and answered my own question out loud.

"…ok, I may have left you hanging about that whole thing with your case but you didn't even have the nerve to tell me about the kid. So what did you expect me to do?"

"I don't know Samone…," he said vexed. "…I just know that I needed you and you couldn't be there for me. Anyway what do you want? You have been saying lately that I'm not concerned about you, so tell me what the deal is."

I exhaled out of irritation, "Well, I just wanted to tell you that the cops were looking for me receive their help regarding Michelle and Tyrone, but I didn't take their offer. I knew that they were going to ask me why they want to kill me?"

"Wait a minute…how do they know that you are wanted by those two?"

"You know the news anchor on channel seven, Janice Carlbright? Well she gave them the news. She told me how Michelle and Tyrone have been planning to kill the both of us for three months now."

"What!?! For real?"

"Yes for real. She took the liberty of reporting them to the cops but the cops don't have anything on them to take them in."

"Well, have you heard from Michelle at all?"

"No, have you heard from Tyrone?"

"Actually, he called me and told me that I'm one dead S.O.B. I asked him why he was doing this after all we been through and he told me that I sounded like a little ole schoolgirl. After all, I do know why he is doing this."

For a split second I pretended to be ignorant, "Why?"

"Isn't it obvious Samone? He wants what I got."

"Well, let him have it," I pleaded. For a minute Joshua was silent; I guess my suggestion was sinking in.

"I'm just tired Samone. I don't know anymore. A part of me wants to get out but the stronger side of me wants to stay in it. But now I have this kid to think about. He could very well be mine…the dates are adding up."

"Does he look like you?" I asked.

"To be honest…he does." I sat up after hearing that.

"Man Joshua. We were supposed to have our firstborn together."

"I know. But I have to accept this shit like a man. I did what I did to make it so now I got to be a man and raise it."

"What does this mean for us Joshua?"

"I don't know. I mean, you will have to accept the mother and the child in our life. It just depends on you Samone. What do you want?"

"Well, to be blunt I want you in my life without any baggage. But I understand you have to take care of your son if he's yours. Let me ask you this though."

"Yeah, what is that?"

"Have you been taking care of him since he has been in world?"

With reluctance he answered, "Yes. She didn't have anyone helping her out at the time and she told me that he was mine. So, I began to give her money. Then she started to get on me about being in the kid's life."

"By the way, what is the kid's name?"

"Jamal."

"Oh, okay. That's a cute name." We were silent on the phone for a couple of minutes.

I was about to hang up when he said, "Samone, I just want you to know that I still want you in my life. But if you choose not to be in mine, well I understand."

I didn't know what to tell him. I haven't really thought about dealing with the other woman and being a stepmom. I never planned on being one. I just knew I would have a firstborn with whomever I was with.

"To tell you the truth Joshua, I don't know what I want right now. If you are wondering…yes I still love you, but this is too much to deal with. I hope you understand it when I say that I have to think about this."

"Of course I understand. Just get back at me with your decision."

"Before we get off the phone. Guess what else Janice told me."

"What?"

"You didn't guess Joshua."

"I'm really not in the mood to play the guessing game."

"Oh. Well, she told me that Michelle has a split personality."

"I believe it. That girl is crazy. It's like she has a mind of a mad woman."

"I know what you mean. Well, I'm not going to keep you any longer."

"Yeah okay, I got to get ready for my next court date, which is tomorrow. Will I see you there?"

"I don't know Joshua. What time does it start?"

"It starts at one in the afternoon."

"Okay, I will see what I can do."

"Well, Samone for what it's worth…I love you and you take care of yourself. I'm here for you and I'm going to make it my job that nothing happens to you."

"Okay Joshua. You take care of yourself too. I will chat with you later."

"Okay. Bye."

"Later."

Time flew by so fast that I didn't notice that it was after seven. Joshua and I use to stay on the phone for hours. Lately though, he has been avoiding the phone. We had actually had a decent dialogue. We didn't raise our voices or have an argument. Even though I was jealous and angry inside because of the fact that it looked like he was a dad to someone else's child, I really admired how he was taking on his responsibilities. More men need to be like him. I tried to imagine how Joshua was with Jamal. I bet the child had everything he ever wanted. Jamal's mother probably got everything she wanted as well. I knew Joshua had the money. I passed the phone up on the counter to go and take my shower, it rung. It seemed like today was the day to call Samone. I decided to wait and see who it was when they left a message on the answering machine. Dedra's short speech was said and then I heard her voice coming from the machine.

"Hello, Samone are you there? Are you awake? If so, pick up the phone."

Her voice sounded as if she was bothered by something and I thought *"Oh God what did Brian do? I hope he didn't tell her anything."*

I was very hesitant to answer the phone, but when I did she said, "Hey Girl," with a smile. Some people say that others can tell when someone is smiling over the phone. I use to not believe that theory but my sister made me a believer today.

"Hey. How is dinner going?"

"Dinner went well and I loved the restaurant. It was so beautiful inside. There was live music and the singer had a magnificent voice. You would have loved it Samone. I'm going to take you there myself one day. But anyway, we are at Brian's right now. He insisted that I called you to make sure you were alright. I remember you telling me that Brian doesn't like you…well forget that. The man wants to help you Samone. He told me that you two had a talk and has settled your differences. I'm so happy to hear that. I want you two to get along since you both are the closet to me besides mama. Let him help you Samone."

"Dedra, you didn't tell him anything did you?"

"Girl you are so afraid of ratting that no good man out. Are you afraid that he will harm you like Michelle and Tyrone wants to? Don't let his words and actions of the past fool you. Move on with your life and let the past be the past." She was right, I needed to let Joshua be someone of the past, but how could I when I needed him.

"No, I'm not afraid that Joshua would do anything to me. And we have too much history for him to even consider something like that."

"Well, why are you so hung up on not telling people what is going on? Let it out."

I exhaled and answered with, "I don't know. I just feel like I would betray him if I did so. I know he is not the most positive person in the world but hey he has been there for me. Besides, he got a little boy to think about. And you still didn't answer my question."

"What did you say? Joshua has a little boy?"

"Yes."

"By whom?"

"I don't know. Joshua didn't tell me."

"How old is this child?" I really didn't want to tell her because I knew she was really going to flip out if she found out he cheated on me, but I couldn't hold it in.

"He is one and a half to two-years-old."

"Wow. That means his ass cheated on you. You all have only been dating about two and half years. Or is it two years? Anyway it doesn't matter. All that matter is that he is not worth keeping. Damn. I can't believe him. You love him so much and he knows this and he still cheated on you. Did he tell you how it happened?"

"Look, Dedra I don't need you to be going and telling Brian all my business. You keep avoiding the question, so I already know you told him some things tonight at dinner. I only wish that you keep this to yourself."

"Damn Samone a'ight, I won't tell him. You are really starting to piss me off with all this "don't tell him" crap. It's getting really old."

I could hear Brian in the background asking her if everything was ok? I shook my head knowing that he was probably standing there listening to every word she said. Who knows they probably had me on speaker.

"Yes Brian, everything is okay Honey."

"Hey, Sista I don't want you to be angry with me. It's just…I'm trying to find my own way out of this without snitching or without dying. So, therefore, I don't want anyone knowing what I know so they can't use it against me."

"I hear you Samone. And for what it's worth I didn't tell Brian anything he didn't already know."

"Baby I just wanted you to see if she was ok…I didn't mean for you to be on the phone with her all night," I heard Brian tell her.

"Okay Baby here I come. Well, Samone I have to go. Are you sure you are alright?"

"Yes Sis I'm okay."

"Alright then...chat with you later okay?"

"Okay." With that there was the dial tone.

I don't know why but a strange case of jealousy came over me. There she was with a man who just earlier told me that he didn't want my sister, but that he wanted me. It didn't make sense to me as to why I was so jealous. My sister was happy and that is what mattered the most. But how could Brian be so fake about the whole situation? On the other hand, he did say that he was split between two sisters. I know how it feels to be split between two, but somehow my love for Joshua was changing. My heart began to sink from thinking about him. From then on I knew that things would not be the same between him and I. I got up from the bar stool and went to the bathroom.

"A nice hot shower is what I needed," I thought to myself.

I got into the tub and began to rub myself down with body wash. It felt good to get rid of all the dirt that accumulated on my body. The hot shower lasted about a good fifteen minutes. Once I was done with my shower I did my usual routine. The lotion was the last trick to my relaxation. I loved feeling soft and smelling good. I put on a t-shirt and shorts then headed back to the living room.

As I was walking toward the front room I noticed that the light had been turned off. I know I left it on. I was certain for that matter. I got a scary feeling about this whole situation, so I ran into my sister's room and locked the door. I guess whoever it was realized that I knew that they were there, for they walked slowly to the back where my sister's bedroom was located.

I heard each footstep that they took. Each step that they took made my heartbeat faster. I ran to the phone beside my sister's bed and dialed 911.

"Yes…," I whispered, "…this is an emergency. Someone is in my home and…"

"Samone…," the creepy voice said through the door.

"I know you in there, open the door for I shoot it down." When the voice said that I knew who it was.

It was my enemy. He tapped the gun on the door and repeated himself.

"Yes please hurry."

"Look, Samone I'm not going to kill you right now. I just want to talk to you about something."

I didn't say a word. I was frozen in my stance. My heart was pounding outside of my chest and my breath was quick and short. I was so afraid that I almost urinated on myself.

"I can hear you breathing Samone. I just want to talk with you…so open the door!" he yelled.

"Tyrone I just called the police and they are on their way," I mouthed to myself. I couldn't get the words to come out.

"So, you don't want to talk, huh?"

He then began to kick on the door till the door burst open. I screamed, for I saw the anger and resentment in his eyes while he clutched on to his gun.

"I'll just make you talk to me."

Tyrone walked into the bedroom and grabbed my hair with one hand. He made me face him till my face was inches from his.

"Look Bitch, you lucky I'm pressed for time right now.…but your man got something I want and I'm going to use you till I get it."

I could feel the heat of his breath upon my face. He used such foul and ugly words describing his feeling toward Joshua and me. It was like he had gone mad.

He forced the gun in my mouth and said, "I ought to kill you right now."

He pulled the trigger back and I thought I was gone for sure. I screamed and he took the gun out of my mouth and hit me over the head with it. I woke up to a paramedic looking at my head.

"Welcome back. How do you feel?" she asked.

"How long was I out?"

"A half an hour. Someone hit you pretty good. You have a slight contusion on the head. Just lay back and relax while I get you ready to go to the hospital." I was just about to lay back, but when she said the hospital I sat back up.

"Oh no, I refuse to go to the hospital. Can't you just but some bandages on my head?"

"I'm sorry to inform you of this but you have to have stitches."

"I understand all that but can't you stitch me up right here?"

The lady paramedic looked me in the eye with concern and said, "Unfortunately I can't. A doctor has to look at you and make sure you don't have a concussion. Let me remind you that you were hit pretty hard. You are lucky no other injuries were made."

As she was finishing her sentence a tall Caucasian man with a beard and mustache approached me. He had curly red hair, blue eyes, and he looked to be in mid-forties. It looked like he worked out for his chest bulged out of his shirt.

"Hello, ma'am my name is Captain Haynes with the Austin Police Department. I'm here to ask you some questions."

I wasn't sure if I was in the mood to answer any questions, for my emotions was unsure as to what to be. First I cried, then laughed, and then exhaled out of frustration. I understood that he was here to help me, but I was close to dying and there was nothing I could do about it. I felt that my thoughts and emotions were really cut to shreds. I didn't know what to feel. So, I just tried to get my composure together.

"Ma'am are you willing to answer question right now?" I looked at him with a dismissal expression.

"Well, I really would like to know what went on, so give me a call when you are willing to talk." He handed me a card then turned his back to me to walk away.

"Captain Haynes," I said, "why did you come here?" He turned back around and faced me.

"Well, Ms. Grey I wanted to help you. I heard your call over the radio and I never forget a voice, so I came over to help you. But since you have rejected my help again I will be on my way."

"Look Captain Haynes, I have just been held up at gun point. The gun was placed in my mouth and he pulled the trigger back. I thought I was gone. You got to understand why I really don't want to talk right now."

"See that's good information you just told me..." He pulled out his notepad and began to write something down. "...just continue. Trust me if you let me help you he won't come back for you. I will be sure to put his ass behind bars. So, do you know who he was?" I was broken and scared, so all my determination of keeping everything a secret went out the door.

"Yes. I know who he is."

"Excuse me Captain Haynes but you will have to finish this discussion at the hospital. The call was made to the hospital and they are waiting on her."

Captain Haynes put his notepad back in his pocket and said, "Samone I will meet you at the hospital."

I shook my head yes to agree with his decision. I was ready now. I was ready to spill the goods. My safety had to come first before Joshua's. He would be alright, I guessed.

Inside the ambulance the paramedic asked me, "Ms. Grey are you alright over there?"

"Not really, I'm very uncomfortable."

"I understand. But it's for your own safety and we are almost at the hospital anyway. Can you hold on a little longer?"

"I guess I have no choice but to do so, right?"

She laughed a little and replied, "Yes, you are right."

I began to cry after thinking about the gun being in my mouth. I had tasted the saltiness from the gun being in my mouth and it was still lingering around. The paramedic grabbed my hand and told me that her name was Sarah.

"I'm here. I know it's hard and that you are in some pain, but you are alive and that is what counts. You have made it through a dangerous episode and you are alive to tell your story. Look, I don't know you, but I feel there is a reason why you were spared. Now you have your life to find out why."

"Thank you Sarah for you kind words…it's just…well, I fear that he will come back. He even told me that he was coming back for me. I just don't know what to do."

"Well, if I were you, I would just let the police handle the case. That Captain Haynes seemed to really care and he wants to help. So my suggestion is that you let him."

"You know what? You are right Sarah. I will let him help me."

After about 15 minutes of listening to her share some of her experiences, she squeezed my hand and said, "Oh goodness…we are here. Let me get you ready."

I could feel the ambulance backing up into the emergency area. The doors to the truck opened and the driver was there helping Sarah get me out. They pushed my stretcher down the long hall and nurses began to help push the bed.

"Yes, this is the contusion to the head," I heard Sarah say.

They then began to talk in the medical language and I lost what it was they were saying.

"Alright. Take care of her and I will see you guys later."

I felt Sarah grab my hand, "You take care of yourself Ms. Grey. Be careful."

"I will…," I said, "…and thank you for your help."

"You are welcome." With that Sarah seemed to disappear in thin air.

The nurses pushed me into an area where there was few people.

"Ms. Grey, Dr. Stewart is going to stitch you up in about 10 minutes. Are you allergic to anything?"

"No, not that I know of."

"Good. We will be right back."

Just as Sarah had left me so did the nurses. I thought they were going to be right back but they didn't show up until the doctor came.

"Good evening Ms. Grey. Are you ready for your stitches?"

"I guess so," I fibbed.

I guess he could tell that I wasn't so excited about getting them, for he laughed and told me that it wouldn't hurt. He took the bandage that Sarah had put on it off.

"Wow...," he exclaimed, "...someone hit you pretty good. But don't worry you are in good hands and you will be good as new."

One of the nurses that were helping in pushing the bed came over to me and said, "A Captain Haynes is here to see you. Would you like to speak to him when the doctor is done."

I was just about to answer her question when Dr. Stewart answered her for me, "She will be pretty out of it. I had to give her some pain medicine."

"Oh okay Dr. Stewart. I will let him know."

She walked away with the same swiftness she had in coming to my bed. I followed her with my eyes and seen Captain Haynes. I saw that he was disappointed with the news. He handed something to her and left. I could feel the medicine kicking in because the room began to spin and I felt lightheaded.

With slurred words I said, "Could someone please call my sister?"

"Don't worry about that now...she has already been notified by Captain Haynes."

"Alright Ms. Grey, try to relax and let me work my magic." I closed my eyes and did as the doctor instructed.

I woke up to find my sister and Brian in the area that was officially mine. They were standing at the edge of my bed talking. It must have been an intense discussion, for my sister looked distressed. Brian looked over my way and our eyes met.

"Look who's awake," he said with a smile.

"My goodness," Dedra said as she walked to my bedside; my sister grabbed my hand and kissed it. "Mama is on her way. You really scared us."

I felt the spot where my head felt cold from the air. It was obvious that they had cut my head bald in that one area. I also felt the stitches.

"How many?"

"How many what Samone?" Brian asked.

"How many stitches?"

"Oh, there are f15...," answered my sister. "...I'm so glad to see that you are still living. A man by the name of Captain Haynes told me over the phone that he held you at gun point."

I pretended not to hear what my sister had just told me. I really didn't want to think about what had happened.

"How long have I been out?" My sister looked at Brian for an answer then back at me.

"Well, we really don't know when you first fell asleep, but we have been here about 45 minutes." Just then my mother entered the small space provided by the hospital.

"Samone. Samone. Baby are you alright? Let me look at you," my mother grabbed my other hand and kissed me on the cheek, "oh my goodness who done this to you? I bet you that no good boyfriend of yours got something to do with this."

"Mama, please. My head is still spinning from the drugs."

"Well, I told you to leave that boy alone."

"Leave who alone?" Joshua said standing behind my mother.

My mother was very startled. She let out a displeasing groan to let Joshua know that she did not approve of his being there. Brian and my sister were shocked to see the disliked figure standing in the same area as them. Joshua must have known that he wasn't liked but he faced the raging wolf and hyenas.

"Joshua," I whispered.

I was even in a state of shock. I couldn't believe that he would show his face knowing that my family didn't like him. Joshua tilted his hat toward my sister and Brian's direction and in return Brian turned his head and my sister looked at me. I knew that got under Joshua's skin because he hated being ignored. After his jaw twitched he exhaled and turned his attention to me.

"Hey Sweet Pea, how are you? You really don't look that good." I laughed.

"I know."

Joshua somehow squeezed past my mother and he was standing right beside me. He bent down and kissed my forehead.

"What are you doing here Joshua?" Dedra asked. My sister caught Joshua off guard with that question.

He grimaced and answered her with a smart remark, "What are you doing here Dedra? I'm here for the same reason you are here. I just regret I couldn't make it here sooner."

My eyes began to roam the room. And for some reason I felt a strange gaze, it was Brian looking at me with discontent. I knew what he was thinking for it was written all over his face. There was nothing I could do to make the situation better. So, he had to just stand there and suck in the preview of how Joshua really was when it came to me. I had to admit the love that I knew Joshua had for me.

Joshua bent down again and whispered, "We need to get a room," in my ear. I let a little laugh flow from my mouth.

"Excuse me Joshua, but I need to get right there," my mother said out of frustration.

I was about to say something to my mother, but my sister squeezed my hand very tight. I looked at her and she had tears in her eyes.

"What is it Dedra?" my mother said.

"Oh, nothing Mother. I'm just so relieved that my sister here is doing fine."

I felt the tension in the air. I looked at Brian and his expression was a pleading one. I wanted to ask her what the two of them were talking about when I awoke, but I was afraid that Brian was going to say that he told her what happened between us earlier. I didn't want Joshua to hear what went on just yet. I wanted to tell him in private. Brian took my sister by the hand and told us to excuse them. My sister reluctantly got up from the chair she was sitting in and followed him out the door.

"What's going on with those two?" my mother said.

"I don't know Mama, but I take it you know Brian?"

"Oh yes Sweetie, I met him when they first started dating."

My mother went to the other side of the bed. She grabbed my hand and looked at Joshua.

"Look here young man…I want you to realize something. This is my baby and she almost died because of you. I don't know how or who did it;

all I know is that you are bad news." Joshua looked at my mother while she spoke to him. I was surprised to see that he didn't interrupt her. "...I want you to leave us now. I want you to leave my daughter alone. Just get out of our lives!" my mother said with stern anger.

"I'm sorry Mrs. Grey, but it is up to Samone. Samone has loving me and I have been loving her. If she wants me to leave then I will, but until I hear those words coming from her then I'm staying right here by her side. I'm sorry you don't like me but I'm in love with your daughter. And just for the record...I had nothing to do with her getting hurt."

I exhaled as loud as I possibly could. The both of them looked at me.

"I'm really sorry that the both of you can't get along, but right now it's not about you...it's about me."

"Yeah, everything is about you...isn't it Samone?" Dedra asked as she entered the designated area.

"Oh no," I thought to myself.

"What are you talking about Dedra?" asked my mother. All eyes were on my sister as tears streamed down her face.

"Since you want to mess up my love life...I'm going to mess up yours..." She turned to face Joshua and told him, "...guess what Brian just told me?..." Joshua's eyes went from her to me and back to her. He had a look of anticipation.

"What?" he asked.

"...he told me that he is split between the two of us. He loves me, but he wants to be with her. How could you?" she said out of disgust.

"Look Dedra, I'm sorry that this had to happen, but it's not my fault. I can't help who want to be with me."

"But you can help who tongue you taste…can't you?" I was certainly shocked that Brian would do such a thing at a time like this.

"Where is Brian?" my mother asked.

"Oh he is gone mother. He couldn't face the fact that her no good boyfriend was here with her."

"No good. No good," Joshua kept repeating himself.

"Okay, okay we all need to just calm down," said my mother.

"Oh, I'm very calm Mrs. Grey. I would just like to let your daughter Dedra know how good of a woman Samone really is. So good of a woman that her own man is willing to forgive and forget. If you were looking for me to get upset with Samone then you will just be looking because I just can't. And the fact that you called me no good just made me realize something…" Joshua let go of my hand and kissed me goodbye.

"You get better and I will see you later." While he was walking out my sister balled up her hand and punched Joshua in the back repeatedly.

She screamed at the top of her lungs, " You stupid…no good…wanna be drug lord…go to hell!"

Nurses ran from different corners of the floor to separate the two. My sister began to kick at Joshua's legs. From what I saw Joshua didn't hit her one time. He shielded himself from the blows with his arms. When the nurses got my sister off of him; he turned to me and blew me a kiss. After that he was gone. I had no clue in what he had realized and why he was on such a mission to leave. Hopefully, he wasn't about to go after Brian. My mother, in her jeans and blouse, left my side to comfort my sister. Dedra relaxed in my mother's arms and cried herself to a point where she just couldn't cry anymore.

Once she was done crying, she walked over to where I was and said, "You are not welcome at my home anymore. And don't ever call me neither."

She grabbed her purse from the chair and exited my little area. My mother was the only one left and she looked as if she were about to leave me. To my surprise I was right.

"I don't know what you were thinking when you decided to kiss on your sister's man but you are definitely wrong for that."

"So you are taking her side Mama?" My mother's back was to me, but she turned around.

"I'm not taking anyone's side. I'm just sticking with the truth."

"But Mama you haven't heard my side. You don't know what happened."

"I know enough." My mother left without hearing my side of the story and it hurt me.

Everyone was just here happy to see me alive and the next thing I knew, everyone was gone. I couldn't believe that I had literally faced death in the eyes and no one was here to help me recover from it. I began to cry big alligator tears.

"Aw, don't cry Samone. You gon' make me cry." I looked through my tears to find Charles standing there with some red roses.

"Oh, Charles you are here," I cried.

I lifted both my arms to motion for him to hug me. He walked over to my bed and gave me a big hug. It felt good and he smelled good, he even looked good. He was starched down with dark blue jeans and had on a nice brown creased shirt. He also owned the latest pair of low cut Timberlands.

Just as he was sitting down in the chair next to my bed, Dr. Stewart walked in.

"Well, Ms. Grey I have good new. You don't have a concussion." He looked around and he was shocked that Charles was the only one who was there.

He walked over to my bed and said," Just let me look at your stitches to make sure there is no leakage." He examined my head and announced that it was his best work.

"So, um doc…wen' will she be able to take em' out?"

"Good question Sir…" Dr. Stewart looked at me and said to me, "…you need to see me in two weeks." I shook my head yes to comply with his orders.

"Well, Ms. Grey you are free to go home."

I was so glad that he told me that. I just wanted to crawl in the bed and curl up under Charles. Charles was the only one who wasn't angry at me. Joshua said he wasn't angry but he stormed out of here like he was.

"Thank you doctor."

"You are welcome. Here are your clothes and shoes. Take care Ms. Grey and call me if you need anything. I left my card in the bag with your items. There is also a prescription in there for pain." Charles and I both shook his hand and he left the small area.

"He seem lik' a nice man."

"Yeah." Charles looked at me.

Charles turned all his attention to me, "Yeah, Samone what is it?"

"I thank you so much for coming. It is really good to see someone who really cares about me." He smiled and those dimples immediately appeared.

"You know I had to see you. When I heard that you were in the hospital, I almost had a heart attack. The reason why I hadn't shown up til' now is cus'…well, I thought you could have had other company." I slowly got out of the bed and began to put on my clothing.

"Well, to tell you the truth, I did have other company."

"Oh yeah, who?" He helped me with my shirt so I wouldn't hit my head.

"Wow. He had to shave that head, huh?"

"Yes, he did. I'm not so happy about it either."

"Well, at least you can cover' it with your other hair."

"You have a point Charles."

"Anyway, so who all was here?" I tied my shoestrings to my tennis shoes.

"…there was my mother, sister, Brian, and Joshua."

"You had a full house, huh?"

"Yep. And I don't want to talk about the reason they left."

"A'ight. You don't have to snap at me. I didn't do anything to you."

He just made me realized what kind of mood I was in. I was angry, hurt, and excited all at once.

"I'm sorry Charles; I really do apologize. It just has been a stressful day."

"I understand. So, are you going to tell me what happened?"

"Sure Charles, I will but not right now. All I want to do is get in the bed and curl up under you." We were headed out the door when I saw Tyrone and Michelle walking toward the entrance.

"Charles!"

"What?"

"Let's get out of here. There is Tyrone and Michelle walking over there." I pointed to the direction where they were.

"You are right. Let's go."

We walked as fast as we could to his car. I happened to look back and was relieved to find that they weren't following us. The last glimpse that I saw of them, they were entering the hospital. Charles had a heavy grip on my hand. He was turning left then right then left again. I almost fainted. It was hard to keep up.

"Com' on Samone. Keep up."

"I could if I didn't feel so dizzy."

We stopped and he said, "We are here."

He opened the car door for me and then jumped in the driver's seat. He started the engine and roared out of the parking lot.

"Slow down Charles, they didn't see us."

"How you know?"

"Because I saw them walk into the hospital."

I guess those reassuring words calmed him down a little bit, for he slowed the vehicle to a decent speed.

"I can't believe they had the nerve to show up at the hospital looking for me."

"You better believe it. That man is on da' hunt for you. And his crazy ass girlfriend is to…"

Charles glanced over at me and asked me, "…well did you receive any more calls from dat' crazy ass girl?"

"No, not yet."

"You say dat' like you specting' her to call you."

"I know it's bound to happen. I just wonder what they was going to do to me in the hospital."

"You already know. Are we going to your place?"

"Yes, I need to get some things from my apartment."

"A'ight." We finally arrived at my apartment 30 minutes later.

"Where is your purse?" Charles asked.

"Aw man, my stuff is at my sister's place."

"We got to go ova' there, huh?"

"Yeah, Charles I'm sorry. I wasn't thinking."

"It's a'ight. Com' on lets go." We were on our way back to the car when I realized I had a spare key.

"Oh yeah, I almost forgot; Ms. Webbs, my next door neighbor has a key to my apartment."

"Dat' ole lady?"

"Yep. Let me go get it."

We turned around and walked to Ms. Webbs door. I knocked on the door three times. Just as we were about to give up I heard a voice through the door.

"Who in the hell is that knocking on my door at this time of night?"

"I'm sorry Ms. Webbs it's me, Samone."

"Samone. Is that you?" She opened the door and she was dressed in her nightgown.

The nightgown was red, white, and blue with stars. It was the American flag as her gown. She was a plumped caramel skinned woman. Her skin was clear of any blemishes and she still had all of her teeth. That's pretty good for a woman that was her age. She told me her age once but I didn't think it was the truth. Ms. Webbs look young, but not as young as she told me. I think she is about in her late 60s.

"I thought I was never going to see you again." I was confused by her remark so; I asked her what she meant.

"Well, there has been some drama around here lately. That girl named…Michelle…I think…was over here with some man yelling through your door. They knocked on my door and asked me have I seen you. I told them that I didn't know where you were." Ms. Webbs invited us in to sit down; we accepted the invitation and took a seat.

"So, when was this?"

"It was yesterday, which was Wednesday. They looked like they were up to no good."

"But why did you say you thought you were never going to see me again," I asked.

"Well, it was just their demeanor. They seemed as if they wanted to harm you." She looked at me confused.

"Samone, I thought you and that girl Michelle were friends. Is everything alright?"

"Ms. Webbs, a lot of things are going on right now. We were friends but apparently the tables have turned and we are no longer friends. It's a long story that I choose not to involve you in."

"Well, whatever the case may be…you need to call the police if you are in some kind of trouble. Where have you been anyway?"

"Oh, I've been at my sister's."

When Ms. Webbs brought up the cops it made me think about Captain Haynes. I wondered why he didn't show his face at the hospital again. I just knew he was going to return.

"Samone. I think we should be heading out." Charles looked over to Ms. Webbs and apologized for the hurriedness.

"Ms. Webb," I said standing, "…could I have that spare key I gave you?"

"Sure thing Baby. Just wait right here let me go and get it." While Ms. Webbs went to get the key I turned my attention to Charles.

"That was really rude Charles."

"I know Sweetheart, but I think we need to be gettin' out of here."

"You got a point, but you still didn't have to rush us off so fast." We were both still whispering when Ms. Webbs made it back in the living room.

"What are you two whispering about?" she asked through a smile.

We both replied at the same time, "Nothing." She grinned.

"Sure you weren't."

She handed me the key, "Now if there is anything else I can do for you…you be sure to call me, okay?"

"Okay Ms. Webbs and thanks a lot."

Charles followed me to the front door. I opened the door and noticed that a light was on in my apartment.

"Charles look," I said pointing.

"I know. I was jus' bout to tell you to look."

"Should we just leave or what?"

"Samone you stay right here. Don't go anywhere. I'm gonna go in." I pulled Charles's arm to hold him back from entering the door.

"I don't think you should go in. Let's just go." Charles smelled the aroma of fear that had settled on my shoulders.

"Look, we got to do this. You were right; we can't just run all the time." I guess he wanted to prove something to me.

Maybe he wanted to prove that he wasn't afraid. But I could tell he didn't want to open that door. He crept to the door like we were on some kind of movie set. I couldn't blame him though; I would have taken longer to reach the door. Charles knocked on the door three times and asked if anybody was there. There was no answer. This time Charles knocked on the door while he turned the doorknob clockwise. He opened it slowly and announced that he was coming in.

"Hello is anyone in here?" Still there was no answer.

He finally got brave enough to completely open the door; and when he did low and behold there was no one in the living room.

"See Samone, there ain't nobody here."

"But Charles, why is this light on? I didn't leave any lights on when I left."

"Maybe a ghost did it," Charles chuckled at his own joke.

"Charles get serious. This is no time to joke around."

I looked around the living room and kitchen to make sure nothing was out of place. To my surprised everything was accounted for and hasn't been moved. I just knew Tyrone and Michelle were going to tear up the place. We were in the living room when we heard footsteps.

"Um Samone, you hear that?"

"Yes I do."

We turned our eyes to face the hallway that led to the bedroom and bathroom. We were really surprised to see Dedra walk into the living room with us. My heart was pounding heavily with shock. I knew Charles was feeling the same thing I was, I seen it in his face.

"Girl, you scared the shit out of me."

"Charles. Whatever," Dedra hissed.

"I'm for real I think I need to go check my under garments on the real." We all laughed.

"Charles you are so silly." My sister gave me a dirty look as she said that.

"Dedra, what are you doing here?"

"Well Samone if you must know...I came by to bring you your things. I also knew Charles was going to be with you so I wanted to see a friendly face. Yeah, me and Charles talked on the phone before he went to visit you in the hospital. Your crap is in the bedroom."

"So you are still angry with me, huh?"

"Hell yeah, I'm furious with you. I can't believe you. Out of all men you had to pick Brian to kiss."

"Just shut up Dedra. You never let me explain anything. There is a logical explanation of what happened. You are really starting to get on my nerves with this whole Brian situation."

My sister looked and Charles and said, "See, I told you Charles. It did happen. So what are you going to do now?"

"I will tell you what I'm gonna do. I'm gonna sit here and listen to this logical explanation that Samone has for this screw up."

Charles set down with Dedra right next to him. All eyes and ears were on me waiting to hear what I had to say.

"Well, first off, I apologize to the both of you for this ever happening. Second, it was a mistake. Last but not least, he kissed me. I was the one who stopped the kiss. You may not believe me but that is what happened." There was silence in the room.

I guess they thought I wasn't finish with my thought for they were just looking at me with eyes that could kill.

When they realized that I was finished Charles opened his mouth to say, "So, dats' all you have to say? Dats' yo' logical explanation?"

"I smell something in here Charles and its bullshit," my sister exclaimed.

My sister stood up from her seat and walked over to me. She leaned her body into a position that looked as if she were about to hit me. I backed up.

"Why are you backing up Samone? I'm not going to hit you, yet. I just wanted to look you in the eye and tell you that you are on my shit list now. And the only way you are going to get off of it is…well, I just don't know right now…" She put her index finger on my forehead and gave my head a push. "…you just better be glad that Brian told me that he kissed you and not the other way around. I just can't believe that you kissed back. What was it that made you do that?" I exhaled and rubbed my forehead on the area where she had pushed it.

"I honestly don't know. I wish I could explain myself better but I can't." I went to sit down next to the quiet one in the room, but he got up from sitting next to me.

"Samone you kno' I love you and would do anythang for you, but dis' is just not you. I didn't believe it when Dedra told me, but now…well I know now dat it is true. Look, you are going to have to give me a betta' explanation of why you did it. Do you want to be wit' him?" Charles face looked as if it had been crushed by a racing motorcycle.

"Charles I promise you that I do not want him. It was just one simple kiss that should have never happened. Remember that he kissed me and I stopped it…" Before I knew it I said some words to him that I thought I would never say to another man. "…I love you too."

I looked at my sister in my peripheral view. She had covered her opened mouth. I took it that my words surprised Charles for he stood there for a minute just looking at me before he came and grabbed me in his arms.

"I knew you did," he whispered in my ear.

"I love you so much Samone. And I forgive you about this mishap."

"Well, I'm about to head out," my sister said with much resentment.

"I can't believe you Charles…you are so weak. You just are going to forgive her that fast?"

Charles turned his attention to my sister and said, "Yes. Just like dat. I am gonna forgive her. You kno' how much I love this woman," with me still in his arms he turned and gave me a kiss on the lips, "why are you so worried bout the way I forgave her?"

"Maybe because I don't want to see you get hurt. My sister here has just proven that she is capable of hurting you. Can't you see that?"

"Hold on wait a minute Dedra. It was a mistake. I said that I was sorry and that it would never happen again. What more can I do?"

"I'm not only talking about the dreadful kiss; I'm also referring to Joshua. You say you love Charles… well what are you going to do about your man?"

"See there you go, sticking your nose in all my business. Let me handle my own affairs. You just handle yours." My sister was getting on my nerves bringing up things in my life that I have yet decided what to do.

So, in spite, I asked Charles something loud enough to where she could hear me, "Charles…did Dedra tell you that Brian wanted to be with me instead of her? He told her at the hospital that he loved her but he wanted to be with me."

After saying that I looked at her to see the results of my spiteful actions. I realized that I had touched some nerves within her. Tears came to her eyes.

"That was so low Samone. I didn't believe you would go that low."

"Well, what do you expect of me Dedra, when all you are doing is bringing up things in my life? You are interrogating me…making me feel low…making me feel bad…so, I had to give you some of your own medicine." Charles let his grip go of me.

He looked at me with a puzzled expression before he said, "You say dat' like you proud of dat. You should be proud dat' I want to be with you." I reached for Charles but he pushed my arms away.

"Charles don't be like that. I just said that to get back at my sister. I'm not thrilled that he prefer to be with me than her. You know why can't we just drop this?"

"We can let dis' go when I say we can. And in fact I want to talk bout it more. You da' one who brought it up anyway, so deal with it."

"Well, look I'm out of here. I don't want to hear anymore lies. And Charles you are crazy if you stay here and listen to more of her bullshit."

My sister grabbed her purse and cell phone from the counter and left. She was so angry that she left the front door open as she exited the door.

"Am I crazy fo' wanting to be with you? Am I crazy for tryin' to listen to you? Make me a believer of what you are saying." I really didn't know what else to say.

"Charles. Okay, I must admit that was wrong of me to say to my sister, but she drove me to that point. I wanted her to hurt just like she made me hurt. I know I made a serious mistake in kissing Brian, but it was only a kiss and nothing more. Brian and I will never be. I have too much going on in my life..." I began to speak out loud personal things that I was thinking. *"...I'm here with a man that I admire and adore, yet and still I'm with someone who loves me very much...well at least I think he does. I can't help but to wonder what will happen next for me. I've been hit across the head with a huge gun and my sister is no longer talking to me. Honestly, I don't know how much more I can take before I blow."*

I sat down on the loveseat; Charles followed my lead and sat down next to me. As he embraced me I began to cry.

"Charles I'm so sorry about the things that are going on right now. I mean that from the bottom of my heart. You have to believe me."

"Don't worry about things. Things will work out just fine. You hear me don't you?" I shook my head yes within his arms.

"Get your things so we can get out of here."

I was about to close the door when Ms. Webb stuck her foot in between the door and the doorpost.

"Samone," she said softly. I opened the door to see Ms. Webb with tears in her eyes.

"Oh my, what is wrong Ms. Webb?"

"May I come in?"

"Please." She entered the door with ease and a slow step.

"Ms. Webb please tell me what's wrong." Before she got any words out she began to cry.

She sobbed as the words began to flow from her lips, "My brother has just….has just…has just been declared dead." I gasped at the horrific news.

Charles stood from his seat and walked over to console Ms. Webb.

"I'm terribly sorry to hear that Ms. Webb. When did this happen? What happened exactly?"

"Samone…just lay off a bit'."

Charles was right. There I was asking all types of questions and haven't hugged or console the woman to the least.

"Forgive my thoughtless actions Ms. Webb." She was still crying but we were able to understand the words that followed the sobs.

"He was held at gun point. Someone stole his wallet and shot him in the chest. They rushed him to the hospital where he later died. The police were able to catch the killer. To my surprise it was a young White male who did the killing. I thought my sister was going to tell me that it was a young Black male, but she didn't. How could this happen? My brother was the youngest in the family and he was doing pretty good for himself. He had stopped drinking and got his life back together." Both Charles and I sat there and listen to her pour her heart out.

"I'm sorry to bring this bad news to you when you have problems of your own. But I have no one else to talk to at this time of night. My family live in Dallas and I'm the only one who lives here in Austin." She burst into tears again and cried in Charles' arms. I felt so sorry for her.

"Y'all listen to me and listen to me good. Life is too short for you to be upset, hate, or never talk to someone who is dear to you. You never know when it is your time to go so, always and I mean always mend things with people whom you care about. My brother and I were close back in the day, but when he became an alcoholic I couldn't take it. I went through a lot with him, and I had stopped talking to him for a while. We were just starting to talk not too long ago. And now he is gone. I can't believe it."

Charles looked at me and gave me the eye that said you better listen to her. I wanted so desperately to change what I did to gain back my sister's trust and respect. What was I to do now? I just know she wasn't going to answer my calls.

"Samone," Ms. Webb said.

"I saw your sister leave from your apartment with tears and an expression with such frustration and pain that it made me feel bad for her. I know you are in hot water with your sister, but there is still hope. You got to continue to apologize for whatever you have done. I hate that you two are going through whatever it is you are going through, but it's not worth losing your sister."

"I do thank you Ms. Webb for your advice. And yes we are going through some troubling times right now. I did do something out of character and it was a mistake that I will never do again."

"Well, Baby you don't have to tell me all of your business. I knew because I heard you all arguing. I didn't hear all that you were saying but I heard your name a lot." I looked from Charles to Ms. Webb and seen that they were both looking at me.

I shied and said, "Oh. Well, hopefully you can overlook this situation Ms. Webb. My sister and I will speak to one another again. If it's the last thing that I do, it will be so."

Ms. Webb took my hand and looked me in the eyes then replied, "That's the best thing I heard you say all night. I really hope that you stick to your word and do it. Well children I think I need to be alone right now. I'm going back to my apartment and I'm going to try and get some rest. To be honest, I think I'm just going to cry myself to sleep. I just can't believe it."

She got up from her seat and walked to the closed door. As she exited the door Charles and I stood up from our seats.

"I think it's time for us to go. Get the rest of your belongings and let's get out of here."

I went to my bedroom to find my bag of clothes was on the bed just as my sister said they were. I began to cry thinking about my sister. I loved her dearly and I hated she was angry with me.

To be continued...

ABOUT THE AUTHOR

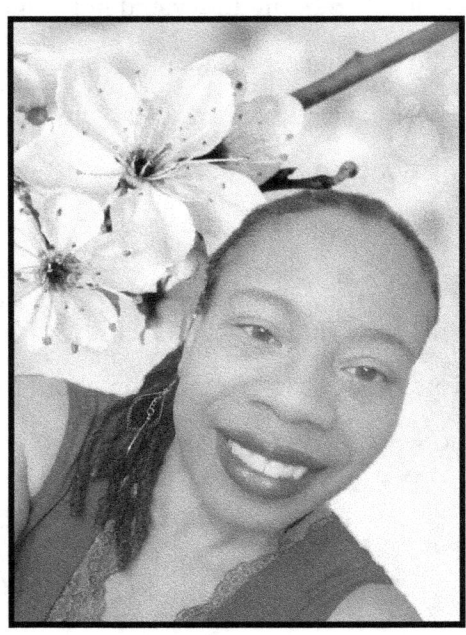

In April of 1981, Monica Betts, aka MoniB was born in Little Rock, Arkansas. As a small girl, her parents divorced and she later moved to Austin, TX, with her mom and siblings. MoniB has an older sister and is the second eldest of three sisters and four brothers.

Growing up in Austin, Texas, in the ghetto is where MoniB first realized her talent in writing. She would write short stories for school assignments, and then be commended on the work. It wasn't until later in life when she realized it was her calling to write.

In 2019, she finished her first manuscript, Love's Mirage. It took much perseverance and dedication to complete the first book of the series.

MoniB now resides in Arlington, Texas, where she writes. She plans to continue writing and give her readers something to talk about for generations to come.

www.ingramcontent.com/pod-product-compliance
Lightning Source LLC
Chambersburg PA
CBHW071824080526
44589CB00012B/907